The Complete Alkaline Diet For Beginners 2019

(Your essential guide to alkaline foods for natural weight loss. Rebalance your PH and reclaim your health with 50+ easy recipes and an all-day plan)

By Leanne Ryan

Copyright and Liability Disclaimer

First Published in 2019.

Copyright © 2019 Leanne Ryan

The author is not a physician or medical professional and offers no suggestions, treatments or medical diagnoses. The information presented herein not intended to diagnose, cure or prevent any disease and it's not supported by a medical license.

The author claims no responsibility to any person for any liability, loss or damage caused or alleged to be caused, directly or indirectly, as a result of the application or interpretation of the information presented herein. Please consult your health care provider for medical advice and treatment.

TABLE OF CONTENTS

CHAPTER 12: 30-Day Meal Plan

CONCLUSION

INTRODUCTION

This book is written on personal needs, where the copyrights are highly secured between the writer and the publisher. The selling of this book in any place is strictly prohibited and severe repercussions might be held upon the entities trying to execute it.

This book serves as a treasure trove for those who want a healthy regime. This book will give authentic details of the definition of alkalinity, the effects of alkalinity on diet and the enormous spree of benefits alkalinity has for the users. In today's world, the diet has become the lingua franca of success and any billionaire can be rich if he gets to adopt a healthy diet. The healthy diet must be focused on the accumulation of minerals, vitamins, proteins, enzymes and together the diet can be used to get all the necessary features of healthiness. This book will give you the insight of alkaline diets in all the formats. There will be breakfast recipes, lunch recipes, dinner recipes, smoothie recipes, and dessert recipes. All these are important to get to the top of the food chain; and being a beginner, this all that you will need for getting a healthy alkaline diet. Also, this book will tell you the gruesome effects acidity has on your body and also, the foods you need to avoid while on a stable diet intake. You must be coherent in your planning and soon this diet will make you fast, fit, and extremely healthy. This book will also explain the role of PH, its definition and how PH can be effective in telling you the reality of a balanced diet. The definition of PH will tell you the nomenclature of all the chemicals that are working in your body. The book tone is very simple and plain, designed to give more value to the substance to the meaning rather than the ideas. At last, there will be the culmination in the creation of a thirty-day meal plan that will help you to elevate your bodies metabolism.

Therefore, it is important that you become aware of this book at the earliest and have a read through it. You will get to know of all the secrets behind a powerful body transformation, you can be the chef of your own kitchen and can easily create, make and eat what you want. You will come up with fantastic ideas that can give more and more value to your body. You can also up-lift your lifestyle in no time. You can also come up with many ideas that can give you a business framework. Yes! You can even start up a business from alkaline foods while reading it. So, do you think that you are lazy and instead want an alkaline state to your body?

Do you think that you can moderate your lifestyle in a good way and have all the advantages of good health? Are you tired of eating grotesque herbs that have no effect on your body and they affect you badly? If yes, then sit on the couch, read this book and eliminate all your jeopardy within seconds.

CHAPTER 1

How does the alkaline diet work?

Are you overweight and looking for a diet plan to help you become lean and fit?

Does your corporate lifestyle hinder your eating habits, and thus, not make you feel very fresh or energetic? Or, do you simply not have the time to research a balanced diet plan?

If any of these questions relate to you, then I believe you are reading the right book at the moment, as this book believes in the quality of a diet, and hence prioritises it over-exercise. The alkaline diet, quite simply, is the answer you have been looking for. The alkaline diet works naturally and is composed of items such as fruit, which have an alkaline

PH value. This value minimises the presence of fat and dairy products and allows you to stay healthy in your daily routine.

But... before we go any further, what exactly is the alkaline diet?

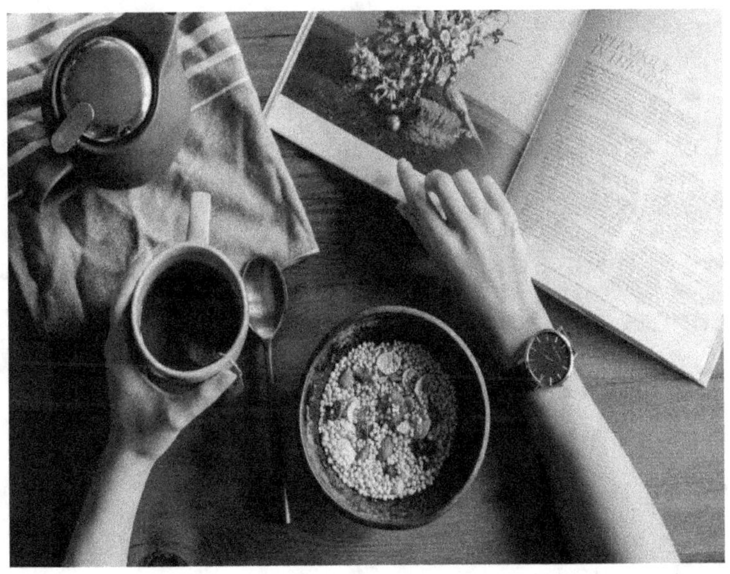

The alkaline diet is a diet consisting of fruits and produce that have a PH value of above seven, and they are all generally water-based in their chemicals. This means that they have enriched quantities of hydrogen and oxygen in them, and hence help to sustain the functioning of the human body. Some examples of the fruits and produce that the alkaline diet contains are: oranges, mangoes, tomatoes, seeds, legumes, and tofu.

In the case of a heavy diet and hectic routine, we always want to be lean and active and if we fill our stomachs with fast food then we cannot be proactive. Hence, we need a diet that is missing all of these fats and lipids, so we can sustain a healthy metabolism throughout our daily routine.

The overall working of the alkaline diet as an implemented routine is very progressive in nature. For example, theory states that the food molecules in an alkaline diet can be so pure in their PH core that they can prevent harmful diseases from occurring in the human body. However, this book will not delve into the controversies surrounding such claims, and will instead focus on advocating the proper use of the alkaline diet for the betterment of the human body.

So, the chemical composition of an alkaline diet is based on both the acidic ash and the alkaline ash, with the latter of the two being produced by fruits and vegetables that are green in colour. The liquid that is used for the synthesis of an alkaline diet is the residue of the citrus food and acts to give a sumptuous touch to the diet.

These two components are produced through various biomechanical experiments that yield potential for the people. Once an alkaline diet is introduced, it used by consumers to prevent illnesses such as kidney stones and heart disease. The fruits, once they are digested, help to make the bodies' metabolism alkaline in a natural way. The diet saves a lot of time, as eating times will be reduced, and moreover, it erases any unnecessary fat that is stored in the body.

Consequently, this could be an easy way to become lean and fit to a lot of people, especially those without any time to exercise. For example, one particular advantage is that it builds a solid muscle mass, making the body healthy and strong, and this healthy body structure can act as a natural defence.

Researchers have also published studies about the diet in the journal "Osteoporosis International", stating that many bodybuilders choose to use the alkaline diet for their own benefit. Moreover, it is beneficial to diseases like diabetes, chronic kidney disease and cardiovascular disease, but also sporting injuries, helping to mend torn muscles.

Once you have changed to an alkaline diet, you will feel very fresh and energetic. The pigments that are present on the upper surface of the foods give comforting digestion in your large intestine, and you will not be able to feel any digestive issues. Thus, in no time, you will be on a clean and balanced diet, where the effects are **natural**, **clean** and **calm** on your body.

CHAPTER 2

Why is the alkaline lifestyle so popular?

First, let us discuss what exactly is meant by a 'lifestyle'? The lifestyle of an individual is based on their daily routine, their calorie intake, their daily processions, and their repute they carry along with them while pursuing their daily lifestyle. For example, the lifestyle of a celebrity can be very famous. He will ride new vehicles; he will look healthy and try his best to do be the best in his movies. He will professionalize his life by working hard and he will adopt a healthy regime in his routine to be successful. Therefore, his daily choices, in terms of food, clothing and routine procession, defines his 'lifestyle'.

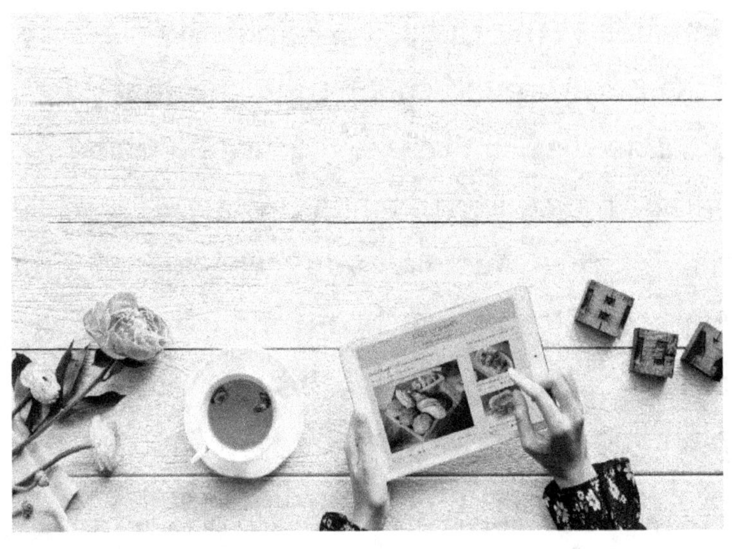

Now, why is the alkaline lifestyle so popular? What basic ingredients does it hold in it that makes it so famous? Well, it's actually because the results of having an alkaline diet are so incredibly successful, and any individual can harness that success and confidence through the mere adoption of the diet. People deem it famous because they become famous or at-least become renowned to the fact that they are in the limelight! The idea of popularity can be assessed through this notion that eating an alkaline diet can make you fit and being fit, can be the source of a healthy lifestyle. While having this lifestyle, you can do a lot of works, a lot of practices and can execute many frameworks through effective planning. This argument can be further prolonged through many different levels of analysis.

The first level of analysis is on the individualistic level. On an individualistic level, individuals get revered to be the lean and muscular figures that have the potential to succeed in life. They can do a lot of things like move composedly in their professional careers, they can focus on their diets and prevent their bodies from being affected by many health diseases like TB, heart cancer, kidney stones and even fractured bones.

They can go to popular lifestyles like the fashion industry and even apply for acting careers. Therefore, on an individualistic level, one can easily transform the credentials of his self into a famous personality. All he needs to do is to have an alkaline diet in his routine.

On a social level, a society steams into the idea of activeness and recognition through an alkaline diet. A society is able to get all the purpose and popularity if it follows an alkaline diet because the functions of society and the correlation of social institutions can be effective in their progress and allowing the intake of an alkaline diet will always open a plethora of opportunities for the society to flourish in the status-quo. Also, the norms and values are equally translated into the successful sustenance of any society and the claws of societal decadence are easily averted. So, on a societal level, there are many features of having an alkaline diet that can be very helpful for a society to boost its formation in the contemporary. All the societies, whether western or eastern, must be allowed to have a taste of this alkaline diet and this diet could be effective for the nourishment of their lifestyles.

The state-level can also be analyzed while discussing the popularity of an alkaline diet. The state is an engine for any countries progress and without its efficient working and statehood; a nation cannot become successful in geopolitics and geo-economics. Leaders need to adopt an alkaline diet system that can be healthy for their country's lead and they can steer the nation's ship with productive body metabolisms. For instance, the food regimen of China's President, Mr.Xi Jinping is of significance. He does not claim to have an alkaline diet but still, his bodily gestures coupled with prudent state policies make him to be a decisive state man. Also, there are many leaders of a state that use such a diet, and hence, due to using this diet, become popular while exhibiting an alkaline lifestyle.

Thus, the modes of working, daily routines and lifestyle are all affected by the proper intake of an alkaline diet. Hence, on a social, individualistic and a state level, the use of an alkaline diet can trigger many bodily changes in the human body and this is all the cause of the popularity of an alkaline diet.

CHAPTER 3

The Definition of PH

PH by definition is assigned to measure the alkalinity or acidity of a solution and its scale usually varies from 0 to 14. The range from 0 to 14 can thus define the alkalinity and acidity of a humans diet. If the PH is lower than 7, then it is acidic in nature, if it is greater than 7, then it is alkaline in nature, and if the PH level is at 7, then it is neutral.

$PH=-log$ [H+], this is the equation used to analyze the concept of PH, and the log is the base for the negative logarithm, which stands for hydrogen ion concentration. The word "PH" is derived from the German words "Potenz Hydrogen", which means power and dominance, and PH value is only accessible in aqueous solution, as such there will be no PH value for vegetable oil, gasoline, and pure alcohol. The international union of pure and applied chemistry has a different definition of PH. According to it, it is based on electrochemical measurements of a standard buffer solution. However, this definition is not taught at all academics because it is quite a hectic one and a lot of institutions, prefer the old definition of PH value.

There are many methods to measure PH value. One of the most important ones can be the use of litmus paper. The litmus paper can be replaced with other colours as well. Like any paper, this can absorb the colour. Most colours can tell the nature of PH, whether it be acidic or alkaline. Also, there can be the mixing of indicators that can provide a colour change over a PH range, which lies between two and ten.

There is also the use of a PH meter for measuring it as well. The inclusion of electrodes is also an essential component for measuring the PH. There is a difference between the magnetic inductions of these electrodes and the chemical released to give the definition of the PH. Hence, the method of pyrolysis is also helpful in providing the measurement of PH. An example of it can be an electrode of silver chloride.

There are many uses of PH, as well. The use of PH is very compatible and adjustable in everyday life and science. It is used in cooking, it is used to design cocktails, it is used in cleaners, and it has a substantial value in food preservation as well. It has its paramount importance in chemistry, physics, biology, oceanography, purification, and sciences.

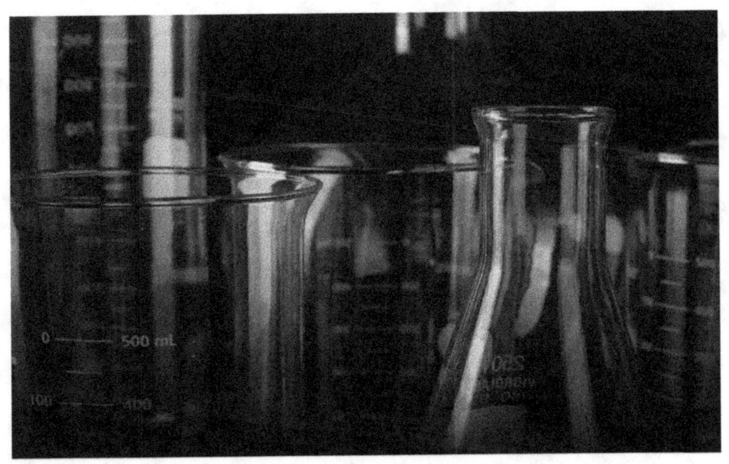

PH indicators are also found in plants as well. The plants that include them are hibiscus, red cabbage, and red wine. The acidity and alkalinity are also assessed in the pigments in plants, thereby allowing the presence of PH stored in it. For the calculation of PH, some charted spreadsheets are also used for the formation.

CHAPTER 4

How does acidity damage your health?

Acidity damages the health of an individual in many ways. The amount of acidic intake creates a PH-less metabolism in the body, which makes for the overly acidic consumption of food.

This means that many diseases can be apparent in the human body if you consume acidic food, and the process of an acidic diet is actually referred to as mild acidosis. Mild acidosis can trigger many unhealthy diseases in the human body. These diseases, along with the acidic intake in the human body damage the creation of white blood cells, which act as a shield to many diseases. The body becomes a donor body, which longs for the acquisition of calcium, magnesium and other vital minerals.

The diseases that occur in the presence of an acidic diet are detailed as cardiovascular damage, which is the most common of all conditions, and it happens in the absence of a PH formulated diet.

When meat and processed chicken pieces are eaten, then the acidity of the body slightly tends to increase. Due to the massive eating habits of these particular diets, the acid released while eating stick to the cores of the body and they are not easily exterminated. What happens is that the severe intake of fats damages and impedes the circulation of blood and hence; as a result, there is an immense gain of body fat. Like this, the outcome of a fat body damages the healthy PH diet.

Diabetes is also a chronic disease, which yields massive sugar accumulation in the body, and it is also because of an acidic diet. A large amount of sugar, in the form of an acidic diet, can be very harmful to the body and reduce the health of an individual to zero. Kidney stones, also a devastating disease, due to the intake of acidic food happens in the human body.

Furthermore, premature ageing also emerges in the human body as the intake of acidity entirely impedes the activeness prevalent in the human body. In this way, the active factor in any health regime is crucially exterminated in the human body, and the body tends to feel weak.

A process also referred to as osteoporosis starts to occur in a human body, too, where weak bones tend to cause hip fractures. As the body is high in acidity, and a lot of acidic intake is still happening due to this reason, the calcium present in the bones starts to decrease. This decreasing of calcium causes the human bones to wreck and crumble. Therefore, human health, due to the intake of an acidic diet causes osteoporosis, which is likely to dampen the overall health of a human body in no time.

Often due to acidity, the body also feels frail and tries its best to recover from any type of bone fracture, but it is not able to recover quickly. This state of the body is known as chronic fatigue, and thus, it is not able to equip the body with the positive energy it needs to heal. The positive energy that maturely transforms the body is not able to be accessed in this case.

Acid reflux also occurs in your body when you eat a lot of acidic foods. Acidic reflux is a condition that is very painful within the stomach and is a condition where the acid of the stomach backfires and tends to cause irritation and damage to the lining of the oesophagus. There is also an exceptional increase in cholesterol levels within the body due to this, and thus, overall health begins to weaken.

These are the real reasons why health tends to decrease in the body. But, there are even more diseases which can be discussed, like for example, heartburn disease, which is also known as the gastroesophageal reflux disease. Drinking a lot of acidic water creates a metabolic rate of burning within the heart region, and due to which the heart reverts water back to the throat.

This process also allows the acid to come back to the oesophagus, and this is actually very dangerous for teeth as well, because it can damage their enamel, too. Not only is it bad for the teeth and throat, but the backing up of the acid to the oesophagus can also systematically burn the lining of the stomach. This lining can lead to the painful inflammation of the oesophagus known as esophagitis. Eventually, this causes the acid to damage the oesophagus more, due to which the organ starts to bleed.

There is also a condition known as Barret's oesophagus, which is very harmful to the body, and it completely eradicates the body's surface, and, due to which, the oesophagus cells begin to become abnormal. This acidity completely narrows the oesophagus, and due to which the storage of food is crucially damaged.

Inflammatory diseases are known as allergies, arthritis, fibromyalgia, psoriasis, and stroke and can be caused by vast amounts of acidic intake. This way, the body level rises to the amount of acidic Intake and becomes unhealthy. According to a study conducted at the University of California, San Francisco, they showed that an average of nine thousand individuals are prone to becoming affected by bone loss due to their massive intake of acidity.

All the body systems, like the digestive system, the inflammatory system, the nervous system, and the mental system, also get severely damaged due to acidity, and again, the health of the body starts to deteriorate. The damaged lining of the oesophagus can also lead to the possibility of strictures all around the body. These strictures are basically impediments caused while eating and drinking food, and they are treated by dilation, which is a tool used to open up the oesophagus.

Consequently, all of these horrible diseases, nasty inflammatory conditions, and the insane amount of damage caused to the organs can all be put down to the outcomes of having an acidic diet. These factors should be bared in mind when thinking about what it is you choose to eat, and what diet it is that you adopt.

Now, we move on to discuss 7 tell-tale signs that show the presence of acidity in your body.

The seven tell-tale signs that your body is Acidic

Here are some of the symptoms related to having an acidic body.

1.   Fatigue or Drowsiness

A possible symptom of acidity in your body is having fatigue. Fatigue refers to the state, in which the muscles of the body get wasted, and there is a lesser chance of activeness within your body. Also, your body is not able to metabolise effectively, and you feel a little drowsy. The condition of drowsiness is a supreme form of laziness, where the body is not able to get active hormones or better bodily health that makes the body more agile.

2.   Shortness of Breath

Your breathing changes rapidly when you are on an acidic diet. The amount of fat intake completely destroys your body metabolism, and you are not able to get the quality of a routine that can be helpful for you. In this way, the breathing changes, which in turn, ends up making you lazy. Thus, this difference in breathing is also a possible way for you to lose your breath.

3.   Confusion

If you are confused and not able to take respiratory processes carefully, then you are likely to be eating too many acidic foods. You may also not be able to make rational decisions properly and have a tremendous amount of brain drain in your body, or you may not be able to give proper time to your daily schedule. Thus, this confused mindset is also a symptom of an acidic diet.

4.   Sleepiness

You are likely to feel very sleepy while you have an acidic diet. You tend to be active and try your best in elevating your energy levels while you are working, but still, minor glimpses of fatigue come. You no doubt just want to just get rid of all the work and sleep all the time! You do not know what to do when a lot of work comes at you, and instead of sorting things out, you become sleepy and do your best in avoiding the task at hand.

5.   Headache

If you are doing a lot of work, you may contract a headache. But if you have a massive acidic diet, then what you don't know is that this headache is likely to return time and time again. You do not think of anything else, but again, your head is pounding like an axe, and you are deemed to be overly dramatic. Receiving a lot of headaches is therefore not good for you, and it is a sign of having an acidic diet.

6.   Jaundice

Jaundice is the yellowing of the skin, and it happens due to a massive acidic diet. The acidic food tends to make all the freshness, apparent on the surface of the skin, disappear, and tries to dampen the fresh colour of the skin as well. Individuals that are eating the diet do not understand at the earliest of symptoms, but they can see these results in the latter. Thus, the emergence of jaundice is the reason why people become affected under an acidic diet.

7.   Increased Heart Rate

The heart rate of the body exceptionally increases when the acidic diet is underuse. The heart rate is instead in a healthy condition when the diet is alkaline in nature but tries to cross its limits when the diet becomes too acidic. The reason for this is because of the acidic intake and the result that the acid produces on the body. The body becomes restless and is not able to be cured under safe conditions, and therefore, it is essential to have a balanced diet, which is not very acidic or alkalne in its nature.

These have been the tell-tale signs that your body is acidic in nature, and these symptoms show how important it is to have a balanced diet in order to avoid such issues at all cost.

Now, a little portion of this chapter will look into the tests that can be taken to check the acidity level of the individual.

How to test your acidity levels

There are numerous tests which can be used to help you check the acidity levels within your body. These are called PH level tests, mechanical tube tests and under systematic tests.

For the purpose of this book, we will discuss the PH test paper so you can accurately measure your own acidity levels.

PH test paper

The steps used for this paper are as follows:

1.   *Obtain PH test paper*

PH test paper has alkaline and acidic ranges enlisted on its front. The below 7 range indicates the acidic range and the above seven range is the alkaline range. This paper can be easily obtained from most of your nearby stores.

2.   *Test in the morning*

This test is conducted in the morning, and it has a two-step flow to it. First, if you get up early in the morning, then before urination get a piece of the PH paper. You can urinate directly on to the paper, or you can dip your penis in the paper and then start to urinate. This first test will be the most valuable, and its result will indicate your PH levels for the morning.

The other step involves rinsing your mouth and using the saliva produced to get the result. First, you need to rinse your mouth with water and spit it out in the sink, before then spitting again. Now you must collect the saliva in a spoon and moisten the paper in the saliva. Note: You must not eat or drink before the test.

3.   *Read the colour of the paper after the test*

The test paper, which has been moistened, will change colour, and this colour indicates the exact state of alkalinity in your body. This range will change from yellow to dark blue. If the number on the paper is below seven, then your urine is acidic in nature. If the number starts to decrease, then the acidity of the urine also starts to drop. The lower the number is, the lower your acidity level is. To have an ideal urine reading, the PH reading should show the reading being between 6.5 and 7.5.

4.   *Reading the acidity of your body*

If you want to read the acidity in a condition that is not prone to error in the acidic range, then you have to change your diet habits. Mostly, people in America have an acidic related diet, and they are meant to have a below seven PH value. Under such circumstances, you can add more vegetables to your diet and can transform yourself with full zeal and courage.

5.   *Monitoring your PH over time*

If you want to monitor your PH over time, then you need to buy a reliable PH chart that can give you proper readings according to your daily intake and you can also save the record for your own benefit. This is the best possible way to keep track of your PH and in doing so; you will be in a position for even better health. Thus, through systematic measures given by a chart, you can reach the summit of your health in no time.

Thus, this has been the framework you should follow for you to get a clear insight into your acidity levels. If you apply them on a daily bases, then surely, you will be receiving updates on your PH level with full zeal, and be in better health due to your increase in your determination to change your life for the better.

CHAPTER 5

What are the amazing benefits of an alkaline diet?

Do you want to be stable in your health regime and eat fresh things too?
Do you think you need to know the proper diet of your regime while both working and sleeping?
If you want to achieve a healthy food routine, then the alkaline diet is the real deal for you! In the previous chapters, we have discussed the alluring idea of an alkaline diet, and now, we will look into the amazing benefits of it.

First and foremost is the sheer activeness that a person tends to achieve while they are eating an alkaline diet. They both feel and look healthy, and they find themselves wanting to do a lot of things! They can think properly and can get rid of inflammatory diseases that can cause them suffering.

Also, they have an increased life span and indeed, it is clear to see that an alkaline diet can do wonders for the individual who sticks to it.

If you want to look fresh-faced, then an alkaline diet can also help in this regard, too. Studies show that the alkaline diet is very popular in making the face look brighter, healthier, and more radiant. There is an extraordinary amount of herbs and breakfast recipes that aid in this purpose, and you're sure to find one you like, and after you do find one, you're sure to soon realise the fantastic benefits that an alkaline diet can have on your looks.

An alkaline diet also protects bone density and muscle mass, as the mineral intake that you get through an alkaline diet can protect your bone density. The bones need certain minerals that are used to cure the excessive number of hurdles one gets while running, and the minerals that are given by the alkaline diet gives you stronger bones for life. If you are a bodybuilder and want to reap the benefits, then you have to accumulate more alkaline foods, and you will soon realise that this will be extremely beneficial for you.

For example, muscle mass can be secured through eating things like almonds and other alkaline foods, and you will have to be very strict in doing so. But, just look on the bright side, and tell yourself every day about the amazing health benefits you're going to get! You will soon feel incredibly productive.

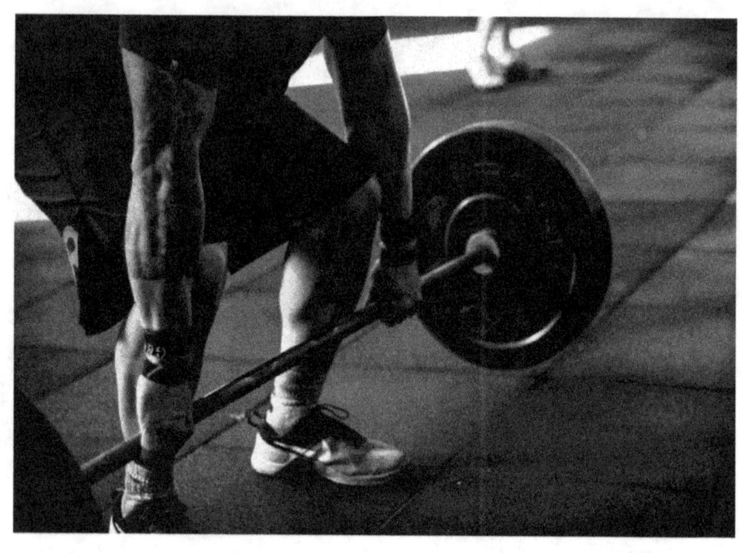

In today's world, everywhere you go, you get a certain level of stress. There is the stress of graduating, the stress of succeeding in life, the stress of getting a job. You believe at first that the stress can be very successive for you and lead you on to good things, but actually, it often turns out to be adverse. Scientists have claimed medical drugs for its cure, but the only reasonable cure is the use of an alkaline diet! The enzymes that you get through vegetables lower the risk of hypertension, and then you can relish in a successful life in absolutely no time at all. Also, your blood level starts to work with full capacity and you will feel like a superman every place you go! Therefore, it is vital you switch to an alkaline diet.

You are also able to get a lot of chronic pains in your body due to many different reasons. You get to the bottom of any problem; you solve it only to end up having chronic pain yet again in your body. Chronic pain refers to any amount of pain in your body, such as a devastating headache. However, the only effective cure for this chronic pain is the alkaline diet. Yes, it is true, the alkaline diet is very important for you to maintain as the blood level minimises when lemon or other alkaline water is introduced into the body. So, this is another benefit of an alkaline diet and it does not matter if you are a walker, a boxer or even a corporate worker, you must have an alkaline diet in you if you wish to have all that you crave!

CHAPTER 6

Alkaline Foods and Supplements

The fruits and foods that fall under the definition of being part of an alkaline diet are discussed in the list below. The list includes foods that are fresh in nature, and are revered to be alkaline.

Detailed lists of foods for you to celebrate and enjoy

The list is as follows:

1. Black and White Pudding

This pudding has a fixed amount of cream in it, and thus it is used in a variety of different desserts, and can even be recreated for many festivals! It is organic and can be created in just a short span of time, and thus, it is incredibly fresh. Many consumers want to have a taste of it once they are done eating their regular meals!

2.   Gingerbread Biscuits

Gingerbread biscuits are widely celebrated in all different parts of the world, and they are eaten with tremendous enjoyment as well! These biscuits tend to be very fresh in their nature, and they are usually consumed daily. Gingerbread biscuits are present in all prices and ranges for the consumers that want to eat them, and hence, they are an extremely affordable addition to your alkaline diet.

3.   Liquor Chocolates

Liquor chocolates are very delicious...many people are looking for something new and want to experience a new flavor. The liquor is actually very fresh for the body, as it quickly gives a fresh tone of digestion.

During holidays, it is essential to have a healthy diet, but sometimes we make some exceptions. In this case, you can eat liquor chocolates to have good digestion!

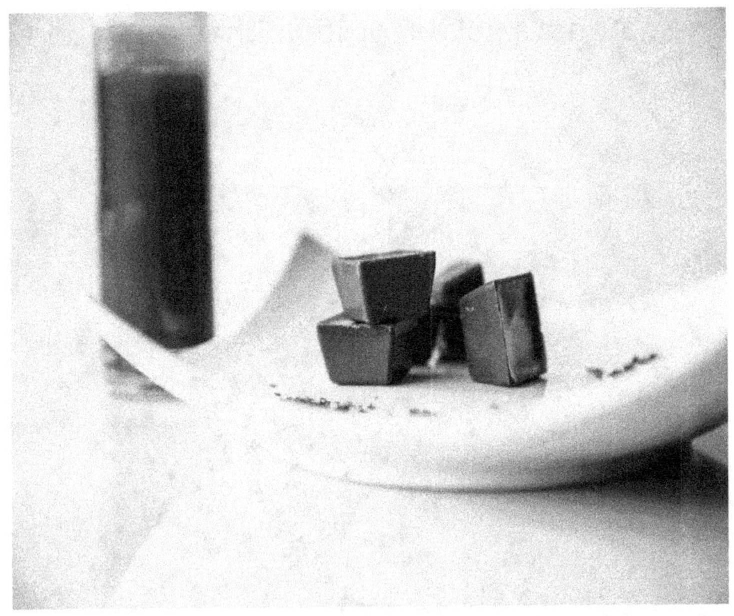

4. Chicken made with a stuffing of fruits and vegetables

Chicken, which is typically made with a lot of acidic strains, can be stuffed with fruits and vegetables, which can then turn it instead very alkaline for the consumer. This process is instead a lot healthier for you and, thus, this recipe is beneficial, as it ensures that you are getting a lot of protein that your body needs.

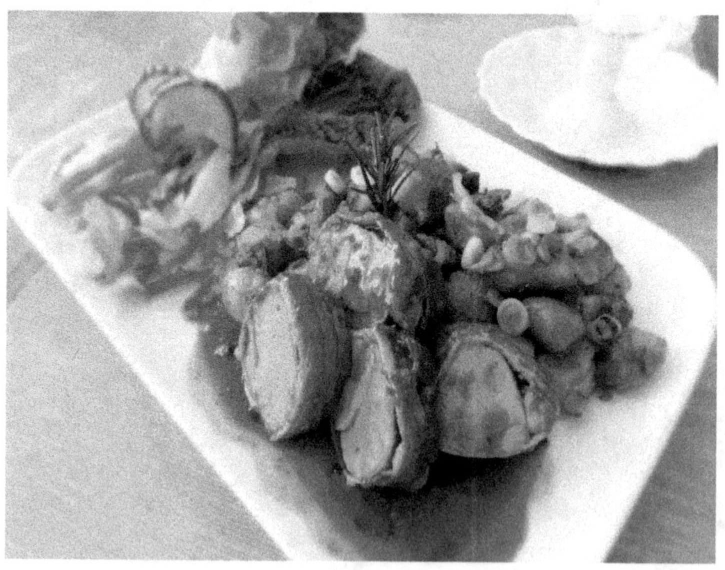

5.   Haggis

This particular food is the stomach of a sheep and it is made by embedding the stomach with oatmeal and offal, and the oatmeal and offal can be hugely beneficial in an alkaline diet, by improving metabolism. This is due to the residue of acidic strains and alkaline inputs that end up giving the consumer a relishing tone when they are digesting it. Plus, as it is made with a great deal of care and intellect, it can moreover be used for many other health benefits, too! This dish available in Scotland, but it is also widely available in other countries and it is therefore highly recommended as a better alternative.

6.   Chinese Soup Dumplings

Chinese Soup Dumplings are revered by doctors to be very helpful in the present age. This popular Asian dish Is a one-pot meal, making cleanup easy. When you eat this fantastic soup the human system becomes very energetic. In this way, this dish can give your body a ginormous amount of help!

A curiosity...a traditional Chinese New Year meal is incomplete without dumplings and a dish of nourishing and soothing Chinese soup!

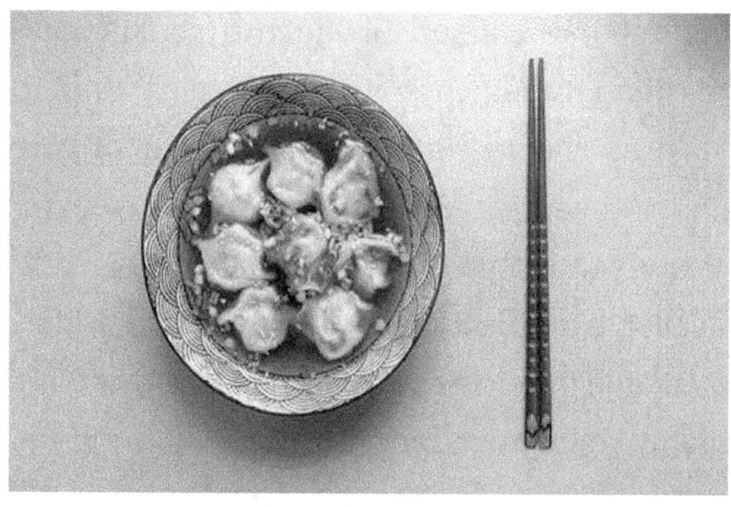

These dumplings are also known as "xiao long bao", a type of Chinese steamed bun from the Jiangnan region, especially associated with Shanghai and Wuxi. Their story begins in the Shanghai suburb of Nanxiang over nearly 150 years ago.

7. Toshikoshi Soba

Toshikoshi Soba is a simple Japanese noodle dish that can efficiently deal with the alkalinity within your body.

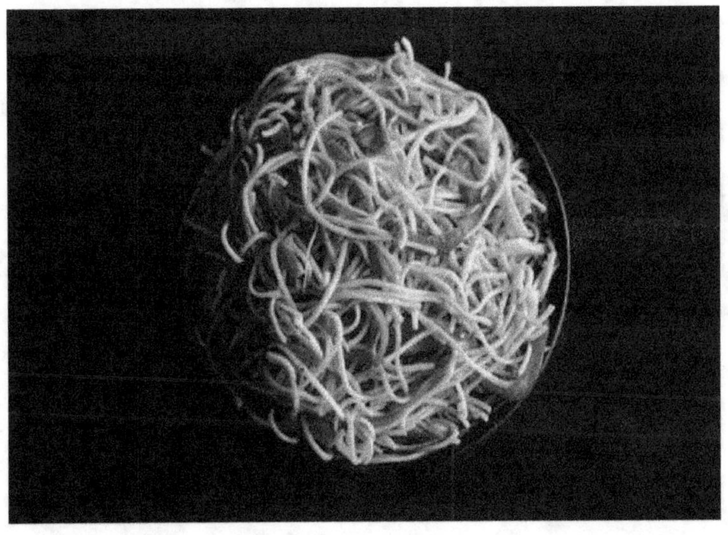

In the Japanese tradition, this dish melts away the hardship of the past year and welcome the journey ahead. Toshikoshi Soba can be very helpful for its consumers. This particular dish is for all the individuals that want a balanced diet, and it has proven to be extremely useful and helpful by the local people that eat it. It is affordable throughout Japan, and the world, and it has all fresh ingredients. This dish is healthy and easy to make...enjoy it!

8.   Classic Potato Latkes

Classic Potato Latkes is a traditional dish from the Jewish cuisine of the Channukka festival, made from shredded potatoes, eggs, onions and salt (it's possible to add matzo meal, flour or breadcrumbs to help bind the ingredients together). If you want more flavor, you can add some herbs and spices.

Latkes are traditionally cooked on Hanukkah, along with other fried foods, to commemorate the miracle of the menorah oil in the Jewish Temple. They can also be made using shredded vegetables (for example zucchini or carrots), sweet potatoes, or even cheese.

9. Puerto Rican Pasteles

Puerto Rican Pasteles is a famous dish that is available in Puerto Rico. Making and serving pasteles at Christmas time is a Puerto Rican tradition. Pasteles are a type of tamale made with pork in adobo sauce*, encased in green banana masa, wrapped in banana leaves, and then boiled. They can be recreated to all different sizes and demands, so why not give them a try?

*Adobo Sauce is made from chili powder, vinegar, sugar, garlic and herbs. This was originally used to flavor and preserve meats and is fantastic in so many Mexican dishes. It's mainly known as the sauce poured over chipotle peppers.

10. Jansson's Temptation

This Swedish dish is very delicious, and it starts with creamy potato and fish gratin. The recipe was first published in 1940 and quickly became established as a classic of the Swedish Christmas dinner table.

This gratin is made with julienned potatoes, onion, "ansjovis" (anchovies or little sprats) and cream. To confuse matters, ansjovis are not really anchovies, but cured sprats! You really can't make this dish with Mediterranean anchovies (also called "Sardeller"), because they are cured differently and are quite spicy and salty. For this reason, you will need to buy a tin of spiced-cured sprats, sold as "skarpsill" in IKEA, or ansjovis (ansjovis have a sweeter, milder taste than Mediterranean anchovies) in specialist Swedish food shops.

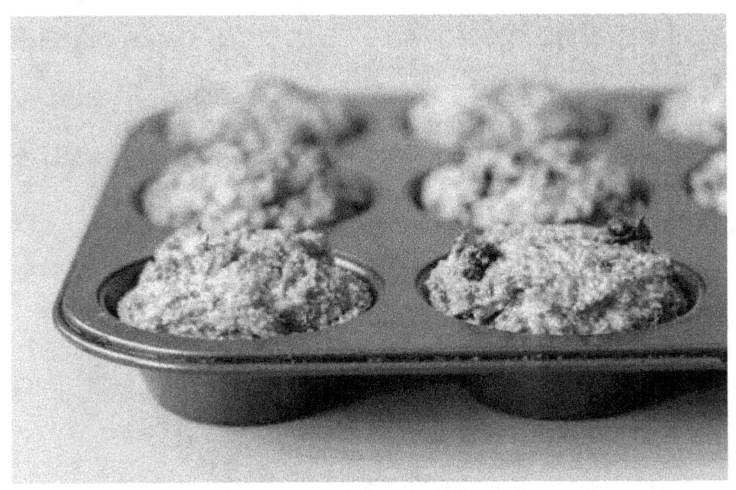

Jansson's Temptation is a tasty recipe that has many positive reviews in its country of origin (Sweden). Now, all you have to do is try it!

11. Traditional British Mince Pie

This dish is of British origin and has its own unique taste. The Mince Pie is a sweet pie, filled with a mixture of dried fruits, sugar, spices and brandy called "mincemeat", that is traditionally served during the Christmas season. The diet of the human body is crucial and must be maintained around holiday times as well, and this mince pie can be the real deal for helping with that! The mince pie has a sweet touch to it that makes the consumer very, very happy!

12. Yebeg Wot

Yebeg Wot, also known as Ethiopian Lamb Stew, is a Christmas dish that has an outstanding reputation worldwide.

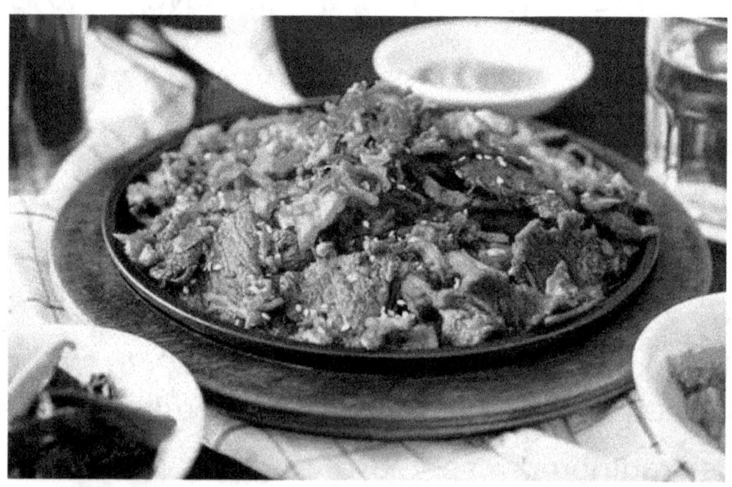

It is made with tender, boneless leg of lamb and is flavored with "awaze sauce", a kicky blend of berbere spices, smoked paprika, lemon juice and wine. This dish can be served with Injera (typical bread from African regions, prepared with teff flour, a cereal originating from the Ethiopian highlands), naan (bread of Indian origin, prepared with yeast and yoghurt), pita or other flatbread (or alternatively rice or couscous).

13. Tamales

Tamales are a typical dish of some Latin American cultures. They are rolls traditionally prepared with a corn-based dough, filled with meat, vegetables, fruit or other ingredients; therefore, they can be salty or sweet, depending on the ingredients that compose them.

14.   Mashed Potatoes

Mashed Potatoes are the last dish of this list. These potatoes have to be boiled and peeled before they are mashed. This recipe is super simple to make with very few ingredients (butter, milk or cream, salt and pepper) and is celebrated in many different parts of the world.

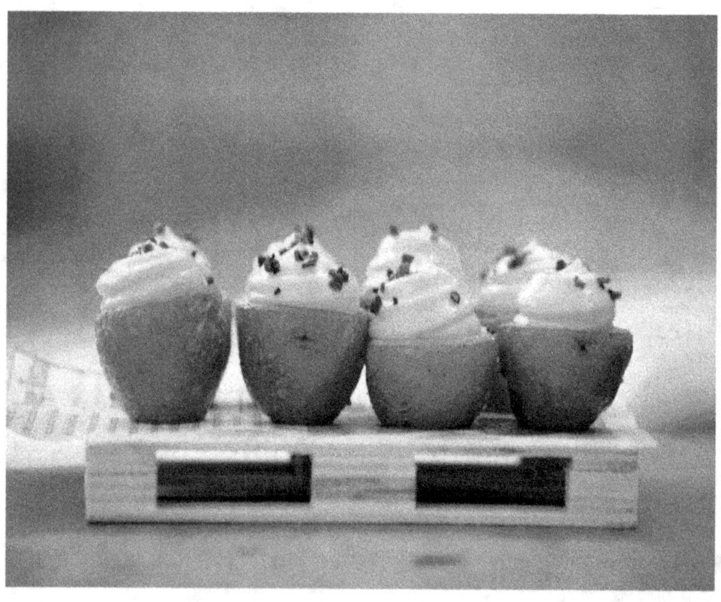

Next, comes a detailed list of foods that you must avoid to be healthy and safe.

Foods that need to be avoided

Where alkaline foods are good for health, and they are likely to be recommended by the doctors, there are many varieties of foods that are not good for your health and it is recommended that you completely cut them out of your daily routine.

With this in mind, below you will find a comprehensive list of all the foods that should be removed from your diet immediately:

1.   Sugary Drinks

Sugar is a dangerous product, it is overly sweet, and at the same time, it can require a lot of sweat to be removed from the body.

Big branded carbonated drinks, such as Pepsi and Coca-Cola, have an insane amount of sugar in them that is too difficult to be removed by the next day, and thus, the human body has to do a lot of gruelling exercises to get rid of them.

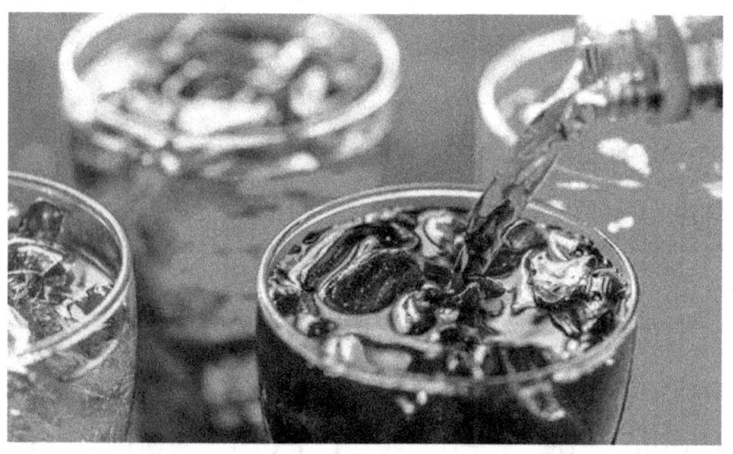

Also, the blood vessels that get in contact with the sugar streamline, and are even prone to collapse, because these sugar particles tend to disturb the vessels themselves. Furthermore, the sugary drinks also disrupt the healthy metabolism of the body, and they make the routine of the body sluggish. Therefore, sugary drinks need to be avoided at all cost to stay healthy and fit.

2. Pizzas

Pizzas contain a high amount of calories and chemical products that can make you overweight and lazy.

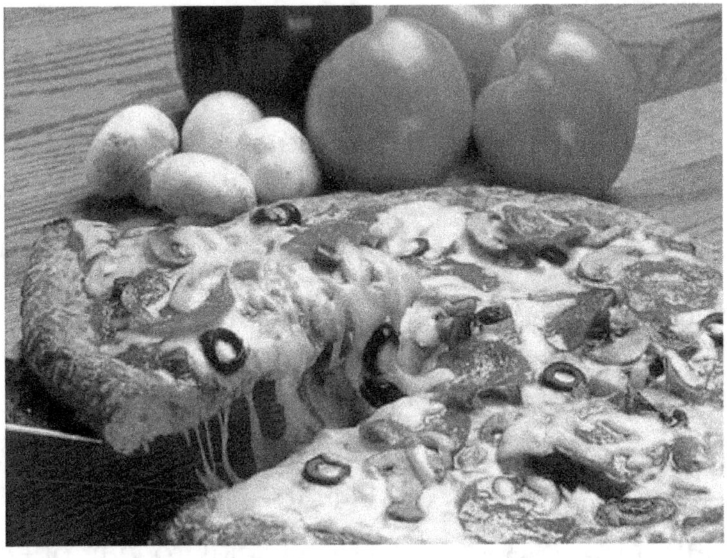

These pizzas always create a source of pleasure at the time for the individuals, but nobody knows what happens to the body after they are digested. The dairy products, the cheese, and the bread can all create a lot of fat that will linger in the body; thus, it is necessary for people to realize the dilemma that fast food creates. Otherwise, the consumption of fast food can be very detrimental to the public.

3.   White Bread

Although white bread is considered to be very healthy for individuals to eat in the morning; it also has some detrimental qualities as well. White bread contains a vicious amount of calories that can raise the blood pressure level of humans.

It is also the real reason behind the vast emergence of heart attacks and strokes in patients. Therefore, it is crucial to eat only the minimum amount of bread in the morning. Also, there is an alternative to this product as well. Brown bread can be used as an alternative as it carries a lesser amount of calories in it.

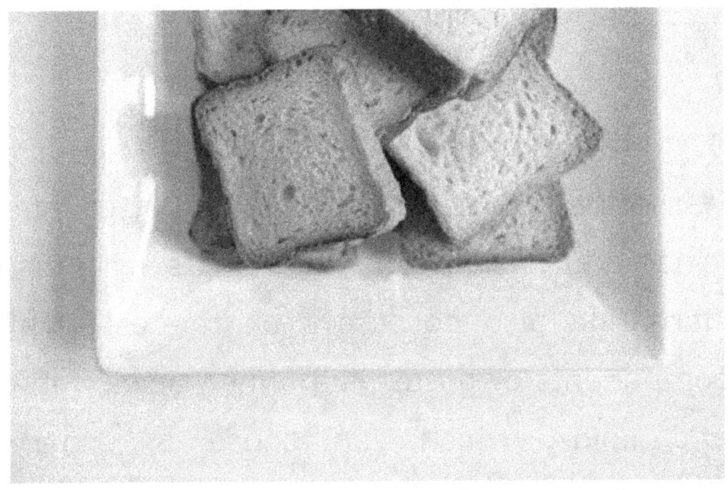

4.   Industrial Vegetable Oils

Industrial vegetable oils are very acidic in nature. They carry a lot of calories and fat oils in them. There are also added fats in them that tend to create a lot of hurdles for the bodies natural metabolism. Their intake can create troubles in blood clotting too, and it can also be the reason for heart attacks. Industrial vegetable oils are very precarious for health, and thus, there needs to be minimum use of vegetable oils for cooking recipes.

5.   Margarine

Margarine is presumed to be like butter, but it has many cancerous ingredients within it. Margarine also possesses all the essential components of butter like amino acids, fats, and lipids, which can cause a urinary infection. It is, therefore, imperative that the use of margarine be minimized at all cost. The alternative to this product can be the use of butter as it has minimum calories in it.

6.   Pastries, cookies, and cakes

We all like to eat a lot of pastries and cookies because we get attached to their delicious smell and taste. They have the variety that qualifies for our interest, and we like to stuff our bellies with a lot of pastries just for that one moment of fun. However, not many people know that these cakes and pastries have extremely high-calorie content! In fact, fewer people know that they create stubborn fat in our bellies that require a lot of effort and exercise to remove. Also, they are the primary reason for a lazy, sluggish routine, and if you continue to consume them, then they will actually reduce the alkalinity of the body.

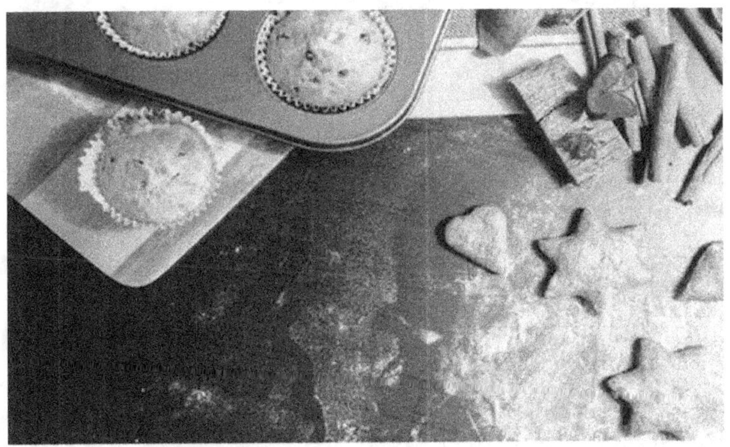

7. French Fries

If you want to become obese in a short span of time or want to win a hefty body competition, then French fries are the answer you are looking for!

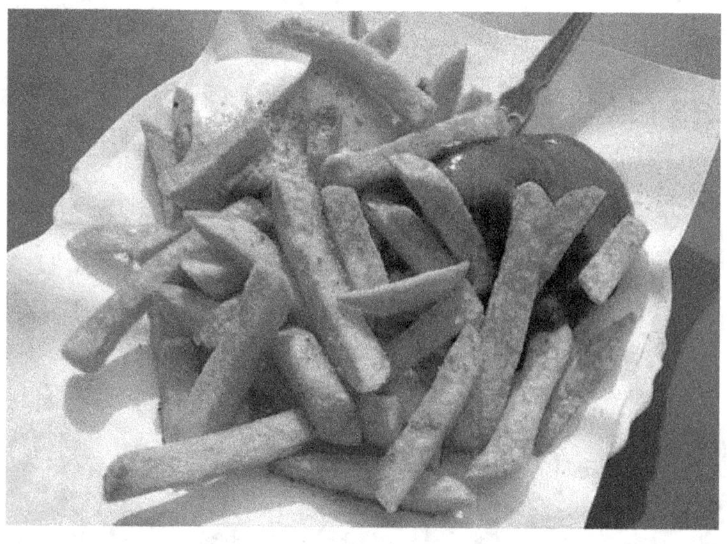

Without their intake, you cannot be fat. Although this statement bestows a connotation that the fries are good, their storage can lead to the rise of many inflammatory diseases in the human body.

They also provide you with a profuse amount of your calorie intake in just one serving, and thus, can make you feel sluggish. The acidity in your body can also rise rapidly, and reach its highest levels!

8.   Agave Nectar

Agave nectar contains a large amount of fructose that can produce a lot of sweetness in your blood. This sweetness can compact your vessels and make your metabolism grow dull and void. Also, kidney failure and other bodily malfunctions can quickly occur within your body, and your overall digestion can deteriorate rapidly. So, you must try and reduce your intake of agave nectar.

9.   Ice cream

Ice cream is used as a dessert for many, but it has a significant amount of calories stored in it. It comes in all different sorts of flavours, and like the other acidic foods mentioned above, it can lead to the storage of fats within your body.

Also, the content that is present below the ice-cream has a considerable number of calories in it and thus, the ice cream is just one big fat creating package for you.

You can make a great alternative to this food menace by creating better ice cream. For creating the better version of ice cream, mature ingredients (without artificial sweeteners) need to be used for better results. For example, you can make a home-made version with organic fruit to have a healthy and tasty recipe!

10.   Candy Bars

If you want to carry a small snack with you that can create a slow metabolism in you, then candy bars are the real menace to be blamed! Designed with just a touch of candy and flavoured with sugar and coated with chocolates; these ingredients reflect the highest amount of acidity in your body. Due to their high amount of calorie content, they create fat storages in you, and they do not let to go away in a jiffy! It is incredibly vital that candy bars are removed from your diet, despite all the temptation of their many different varieties, as their intake can damage your cholesterol level as well.

11.   Processed Meat

Meat has the highest amount of protein than any other food. However, processed meat needs to be removed from your diet by any means possible, because it has all the chemical ingredients necessary to trigger fat accumulation in your body that it is damaging to the human metabolism. It is also not covered in good packing, and it gives a sheer amount of negativity in your body as well. The meat further destroys the excellent quality of chlorine in your body, and you are not able to regain the advantages of a balanced diet sensibly.

12. Processed Cheese

Processed cheese is filled with filler ingredients that completely eradicate protein and healthy fats within your body. On the contrary, regular cheese is excellent for the body as the content of the food is compatible with your body. Therefore, processed cheese is not suitable for your body as it destroys the healthy metabolism of the body.

13. Packaged Turkey

Turkey has an abundance of sodium and proteins in it, but packaged turkeys are not able to provide you with the balanced diet you crave. Its packaging is also very detrimental to your health. You should ideally buy packages with less sodium, or you may end up being lazy and feel very unhealthy. Thus, packaged turkey is part of a 'good' diet but is not part of an alkaline diet, and you should probably be removed.

14.   Energy Bars

These energy bars are hailed to be 'energy' bars, but you are not able to achieve a full energy diet because of them.

The energy bars are not able to give the critical intake of proteins as well and, according to Dr.Garwis, protein bars are all just processed chemicals!

These little chemical creations do absolutely nothing to benefit your health, and they do not help you maintain a good metabolism rate.

15. Packed Bran Muffins

This recipe can serve as a quick breakfast, but actually, it gives you a lot of calories in doing so! It has an insane amount of chemicals and sugar, formaldehyde, wheat, and flour, and they all try their best to creating fat!

16. Multigrain Bread

This bread has the sugar embedded chemical in it that can be harmful to your body if you consume a lot of it.

It is assumed to be very healthy as it has a multi-grain fibre attached to it, but overall, it has a lot of wheat and sugar in it, which can be detrimental for your health. It can also cause a spike in your blood sugar level, and you will likely feel remorseful while you are eating it.

17. Flavoured Oatmeal

Well, do you think that you can find any faults in regular oatmeal when it is served in front of you? It seems to have everything that the body requires, right? However, research has proven that oatmeal tends to contain an insane amount of calories, and it has a lot of sodium and sugar-related chemicals. Also, the creamy flavour promotes fats and chemicals in yourself and thus can be very dangerous for your health and wellbeing!

18. Couscous

Although couscous looks like a grain, it's actually pasta. Couscous wants to build the massive intake of alkalinity in you; however, the sugar and sodium level in couscous is very high, and at some level, it can be very dangerous for your health as well.

As you can see, these foods are not suitable for the body as they discourage the healthy workings of the body and try to impede your natural metabolism. The damage that these ingredients cause to our bodies is obscene, and thus, we must use and consume super-foods, which can heal the body with full zeal.

Super-foods that can heal the body

Following are some of the foods that can heal your body in no time.

1.   Kelp

Kelp is a portion of fresh green food that boosts iodine intake within the body. It is also rich in calcium, magnesium, and potassium, which can all be very supplemental for the body. The consumption of kelp should be very moderate to help to give the body better control over its overall care. The green ingredients reduce fat and terrible amino acids that could be harmful to the body, while also, the love handles that are created on the sides of the stomach are easily rectified with full zeal and energy.

2.   Ginger

Ginger is beneficial in treating arthritis and can be very fitting for aiding in healthy digestion as well. It is recognized worldwide for its ability to treat nausea, and it has been doing it spectacularly!

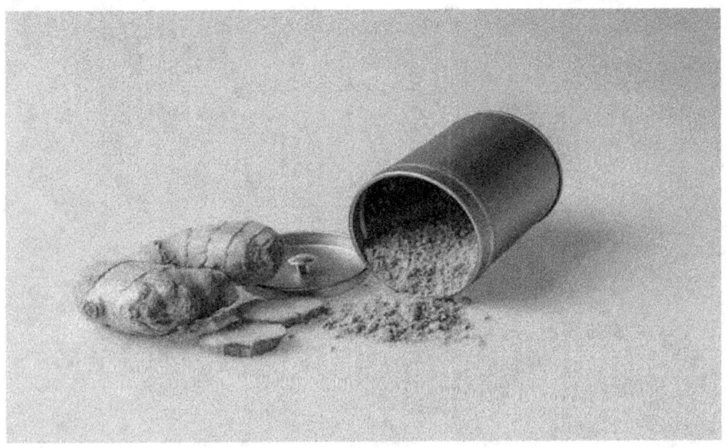

3. Mushrooms

Many types of mushrooms can cater to healthy digestion in the body. The types include a white button, shiitake, portabella, and cremini. These mushrooms also lower the cholesterol level in the body and create an alkaline state of digestion. These mushrooms are easy to cook and eat, and as well as their healing benefits, they can be used in desserts as well!

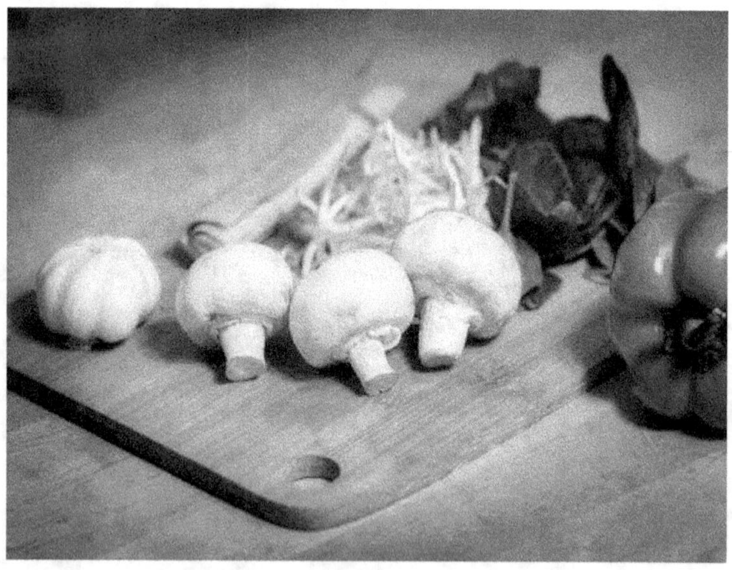

4.   Beetroot

Beets contain a plethora of supplements for the body. They give carbs, calcium, iron, vitamin A and vitamin C. These vitamins are beneficial for the body as they help to regenerate a lot of energy which is needed for day to day life. Many people in the contemporary world are pursuing beets, simply for the gain of more carbohydrates. Better yet, beets are easy to buy and afford and give outstanding performances in aiding the natural processes of the human body.

5.   Probiotics

What exactly are probiotics? Probiotics are the microorganisms that attack germs entering your body, and they are instrumental in making you free of diseases. They are very tiny in their chemistry and can be found in yoghurt, kefir and soy beverages. These probiotics can also be obtained in many other products as well. These probiotics can be used to treat irritable bowel syndrome, skin infections, and certain cancers.

6.   Swiss Chard

This chard provides you with a tremendous source of vitamins C, E and K. It also gives you lots of fibre, zinc, and calcium! The chard is also available in a variety of leaf colours, and its taste is a combination of both salty and bitter. This nutrition-packed vegetable supports bone health; fights stress-related diseases and also fights anti-inflammatory diseases.

7.   Aloe Vera

Aloe Vera is a curing herb that is used to heal facial scars and also caters to digestion issues in the body. These digestion issues are due to an acidic diet creating burning conditions in the body, such as heartburn, and the intake of aloe vera can also provide healthy minerals. It is found in almost every price and in lots of different varieties. It is anti-inflammatory in nature, and it attacks all the inflammatory diseases that can be dangerous for the body.

Within the core of Aloe Vera is a bio-mediating form that promotes overall good health and aids in this process. It can do this because it has all the chemical ingredients that can generate sustenance for the entire human system! Moreover, the herb specialises in curing headaches and tries its best to create a more balanced form within the body. Therefore, aloe vera is a particularly healthy herb that is extremely helpful in aiding in the bodies natural recovery.

In a spiritual sense, there are also spiritual lessons to be learnt from the use of Aloe Vera as well. The herb relaxes the mental coordination system within the human body and the human being who is taking the herb, thus allowing them to come into an emotional connection with the herb. The herb transcends its healing qualities to the human at all cost, and there is no interference with its extraction.

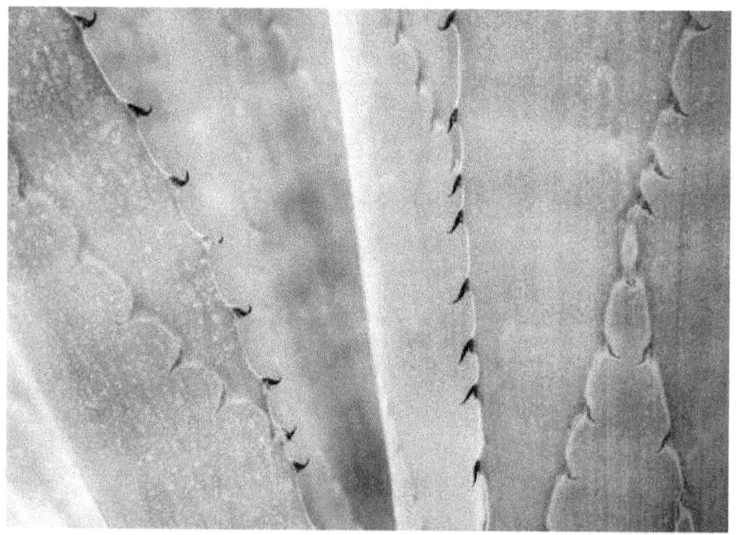

8.   Apple Cider Vinegar

Apple Cider Vinegar is a curing herb that gives a lot of relaxation to the human body. It has a lot of very efficient probiotics that can cure the mindset of a tensed human body, and it can also generate precise salvation to the human body as well!

9.   Lemons

Lemons are very beneficial for human metabolism.

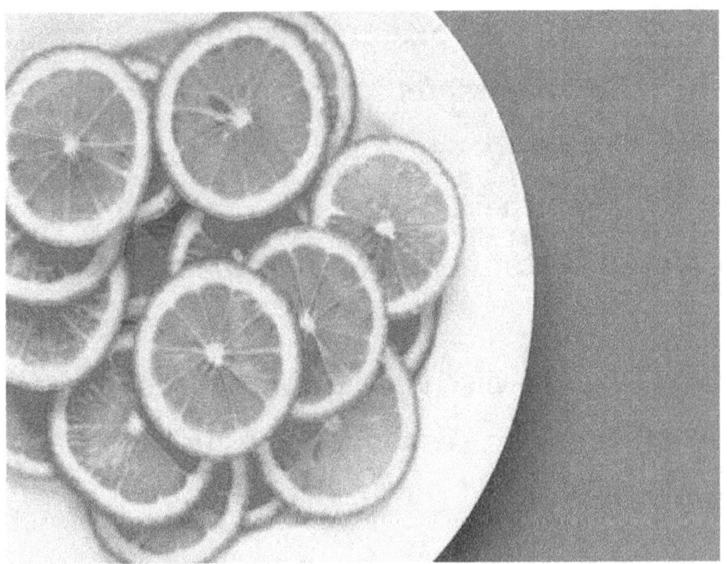

They have enriched zinc components in them that help to carve a spectacular body! With the consumption of lemons, digestion becomes very easy, and there is no regurgitation back into the oesophagus. Throat scratches and burns can also be quickly healed using lemonade, and thus, lemons are a fantastic all-round package, and are highly recommended!

These are the so-termed 'superfoods' that could be very useful for people in the longer run. These foods are readily available in every supermarket, and they can be used to harness better health and wellbeing!

Next, we will discuss the role of fresh herbs, which can be essential in curing health problems.

The role that fresh herbs play in improving health

For better health, the consumption of specific food ingredients is significant. Since the medieval era, the use of herbs has garnered a lot of attention, and the people that consume a lot of them are always in good shape and mood. Herbs add the right amount of flavour to the food, and they can give a fruitful result in the human conscience as well.

There is a feature present in herbs, known as the protective polyphenols. These phenols specialize in protecting the body from inflammatory diseases, and they can be very effective in their use. The herbs can also do their best in exterminating the germs prevalent in your mind and by dint of their freshness; the herbs can take you to many places of quality.

So, the role of fresh herbs is to make your body good and enhance your systems overall, so if you can find any of these herbs in any of the local food stores near you, then you should definitely pick them up!

There are many herbs like Parsley, Tarragon, Basil and Thyme that can provide many protecting hormones. Therefore, it is vital that these fresh herbs can be adapted into our daily lifestyles, and there should not be an issue with eating them.

The herb of *rosemary* can be very useful for mental coordination and memory. It has green pigments that can refresh the medulla neurons for the day, and thus, within a day; for example, one could recall all the important statistics for academia and professional contracts.

For ladies, the herb *parsley* can be very fundamental as it cures breast cancer, which is a terrible disease. Many doctors that are the prodigies of their careers recommend the strenuous use of this herb and many consumers today still support its use. The purpose of this herb has been thoroughly studied by scientists over the years, and there has been no issue about its chemistry. Also, the use of this herb is effortless, and thus, it should not be ignored at any cost in your daily life.

Peppermint is an incredible herb that has many potential uses. It is used by patients, who have burning digestion and it is used to soothe your entire colon and other fibre reflexes. Also, the amount of fat accumulation that you have in your body is lowered to a minimum by its use, and it is recommended by doctors to their patients who have inflammatory diseases.

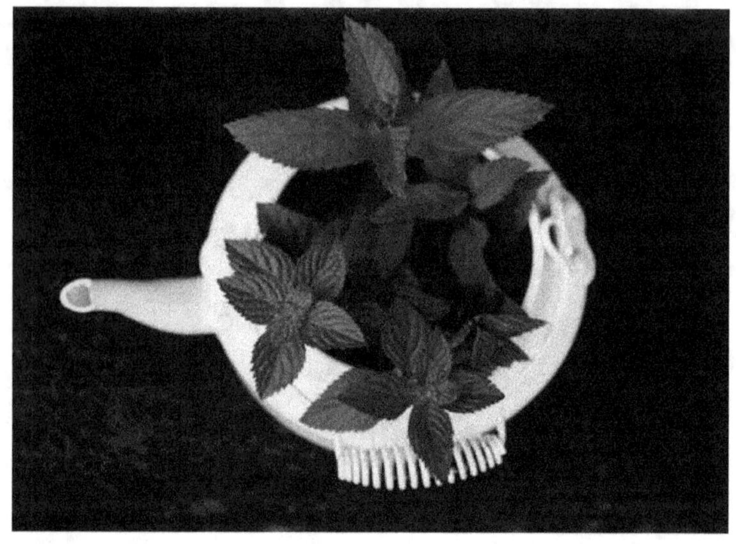

Oregano is, however, the best and most suitable herb that can fight with inflammatory diseases.

Often there are acidic diets that cause inflammation in your body and to find total relaxation within your body, you require a herb that is capable of extinguishing the heat in your body. This herb has all the capabilities needed for this process, and it is recommended by many doctors! Thus, oregano is the real deal for you if you tend to be inflicted with inflammation a lot of the time in your daily life.

Fresh thyme can kill all the intoxicants within your body that become a part of your daily routine. However, if you are not able to get the real deal through your eating habits, then you just have to try this fresh thyme! This herb, when eaten, can kill all the intoxicated pigments that come into contact with your red blood cells. If you are not able to get the result from a drug, which you intended to use instead of this herb, then the only possible way for you to get to the glory of better health is the authentic use of this herb.

Therefore, it is recommended that you do not quiver with fear while you try it, but you eat it with all the interest of bettering your overall health.

Another herb that comes to mind when there is a discussion about the role of herbs is *cinnamon*. Cinnamon is a herb traditionally used by many ancient cultures. It is indicated for gastrointestinal problems, urinary infections, relieving symptoms of colds and flu and has remarkable anti-fungal and anti-bacterial properties.

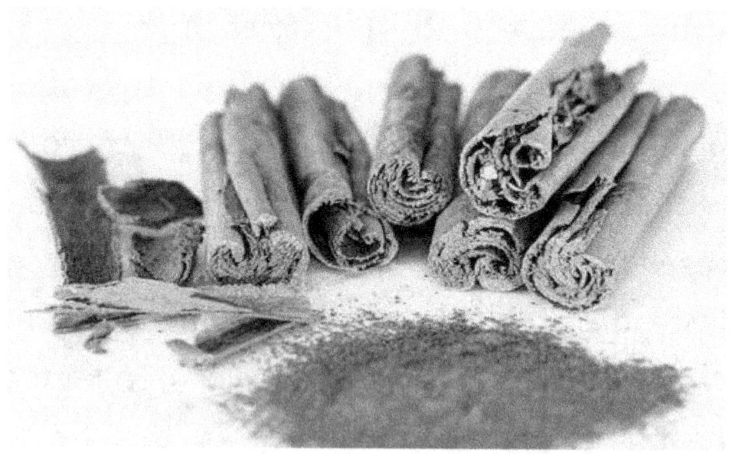

It has a chemical product in it known as the underlined cinnamaldehyde, and that caters to the inflammatory influx of a variety of different diseases. It also lowers the sugar levels in your body (some studies have shown that Cinnamon helps people with diabetes metabolise sugar better) and gives you an energizing boost to your daily routine!

There is a herb, which improves brain memory and the neuron's transmission throughout the body, and that herb is *sage*.

In fact, in the medieval era, it was hailed to be the ultimate healing product. It is a herb, which can be acquired in any way throughout the globe, and it plays the critical role of a doctoring tool within the body.

Acetylcholine is a drug that is present in the hindbrain of the body, and its profuse presence can dampen the thinking process as well. Thus, the use of this herb can finally lead to healthy, better working metabolism.

If you are infected and want to get rid of all the diseases that are clawing your body then the herb, *holy basil* could be useful for you. The bacteria and germs that are on your food and hence meet in your body can be exterminated by the mere consumption of this herb. The immune system, which is a guarding system for your body, can also be enhanced by this herb, and it is used with full zeal by all the users.

To fight the menace of cancer, many herbs can be used. *Cayenne Pepper* is a herb that is attributed to this property. It contains a specific chemical in it that burns a massive amount of fat promptly.

That chemical is <u>capsaicin</u>, which is typically an organic drug that can help to reduce fat storage and thus the body begins to work more effectively (the capsaicin in cayenne peppers has metabolism-boosting properties).

Apart from these characteristics, cayenne also returns good face colour and aids in returning proper digestion to the body as well (may aid digestive health). According to a study, conducted in America, three per cent of the public, use cayenne for rapid fat loss. Thus, this drug can do a lot to prevent body disorders (may lower blood pressure and eliminate migraines).

Fenugreek is a fresh herb that improves blood sugar level control. In our body, sugar levels oscillate between many numbers, and to have a healthy number, a fresh herb is required. One gram of fenugreek can lower one gram of sugar level in the body!

Herbs can also help to regulate bowel movements. Irregular bowel movements are a movement that is created by lousy blood regulation in the body.

Herbs can reduce the risk of irregular bowel movements, and moreover, can fix the temperature of the body with full zeal and determination!

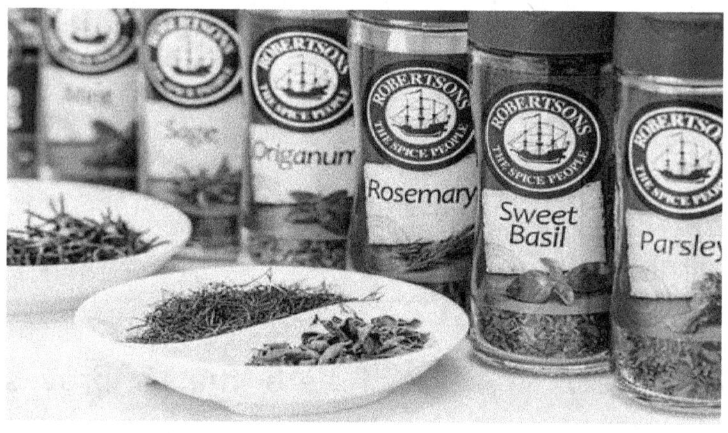

Therefore, the description mentioned above clearly indicates the pivotal role that herbs play in creating a healthy regime within a human's body. The use of herbs is highly encouraged by many different medical departments, and thus, individuals should be motivated to use them with full courage.

Now, attention will be given to alkalizing and healing supplements. Alkalizing has been briefly described in the previous chapters, and it is essential to see which of the supplements can do the alkalizing in a fixed amount of time.

Alkalizing and healing supplements

The alkaline diet has many tremendous health benefits. For example, it improves bone density and increases muscle mass, and it provides a guard against inflammation. Additionally, the body is also able to lower the effects of chronic pain on an alkaline diet. Moreover, there is a lower risk for hypertension or having a stroke while a person is on an alkaline diet. This is because of the vitamin absorption in the body from all the alkaline foods, and thus, there is a higher magnesium accumulation in the body, and this improves the overall immune system of the body, acting as a protective barrier against diseases such as things like cancer.

One can hence improve the overall health and increase the protection against harmful diseases by implementing some of these vital supplements below into the daily routine. These supplements will aid in giving you an alkaline diet:

1.   Tomatoes

Tomatoes are the best alkaline foods that you can possibly have as they have many nutrients in them, and they are also a great source of Vitamin C. They also provide you with a great deal of Vitamin B6. You can have a tomato by itself, or you can choose to use it in your favourite salad as well! Therefore, it is an enriched supplement that provides you with an alkaline diet. In addition, tomatoes contain lycopene, which can help to prevent heart attacks.

2.   Almonds

If you want to have a quick alkaline supplement, then almonds could be your best choice! They are composed of a high amount of fat, which can easily be used to store a fantastic amount of energy in you for when you need it most!

3.   Spinach

This leafy vegetable, which is green in colour, is fantastic for your health. The chlorophyll contained in the green pigment is pure sunlight energy and highly alkalizing to our bodies. It is most beneficial eaten raw, in salads or even juiced with some other alkaline foods. If you want a fresh alkaline meal, then spinach is the real deal for you!

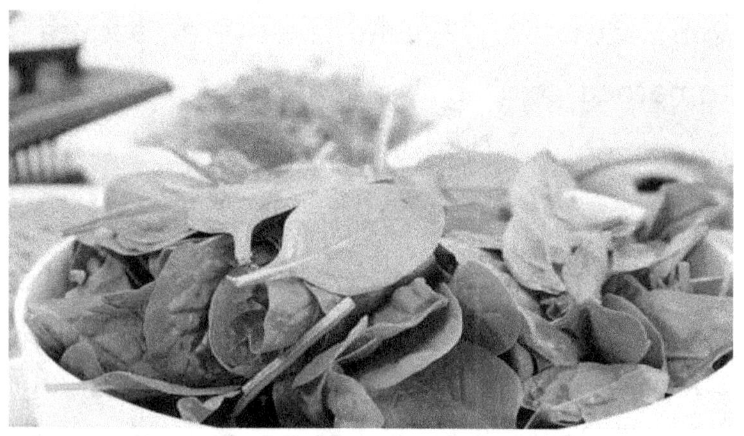

4. Parsley

Parsley is a food that is rich in alkalinity and has the bonus of being able to be used for a variety of different purposes. It can be used to cleanse the kidneys, or it can be used to curb the heat from poor digestion, like heartburn. You can also use it in a variety of different ways to make your food look good!

5.   Jalapeno

For a healthy alkaline diet, the jalapeno is crucial. Jalapenos can be used in many ways, and this alkaline supplement can support the endocrine system as well.

6.   Avocado

If you are a bodybuilder and you want to become the next big bodybuilding star in the world, then you just have to try avocado!

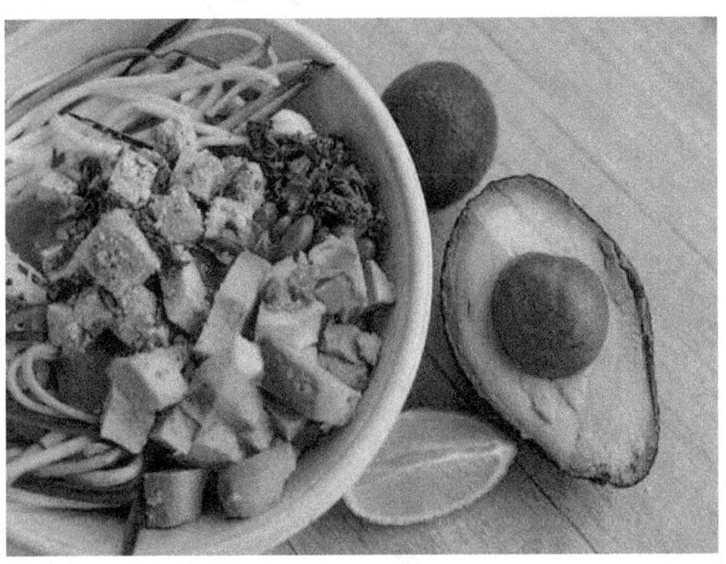

This supplement is an absolute powerhouse, and if you use it properly, then you will undoubtedly achieve all the levels healthiness and agility you want!

Avocado is also packed full of essential omega oils, for a healthy heart and great skin, hair and nails, as well as maintaining good joint functionality.

7. Basil

Basil is a fantastic alkaline supplement that is designed to boost energy levels. It is composed of a scientific chain of carbohydrates that ensures anti-inflammation. It is available worldwide in most shops, and it is incredibly easy to eat.

It is incredibly important to maintain an alkaline state, so the supplement basil should be consumed regularly.

8.   Dark Lettuces

If you think that you will be missing the fantastic dark lettuces from your alkaline diet, then you are sorely mistaken! You have to try this ingredient as it will have enormous health benefits, but to reap these benefits, you must understand how it works. It has a deep colour because of the minerals in it and that colour indicates the presence of special vitamins, like vitamin C and vitamin K. The green pigment includes chlorophyllin and this can cause you to feel very fresh and energized in your daily routine!

9.   Celery

This is an excellent alkalizing food for many different reasons. It has a vast amount of water in it, zero calories, and it also has vitamins C and K. Its composition is filled with electrolytes that can provide better health to your body in no time at all, and can even reduce high blood pressure. It's important to remember that cooking destroys some of the vitamins and minerals and makes it less alkaline.

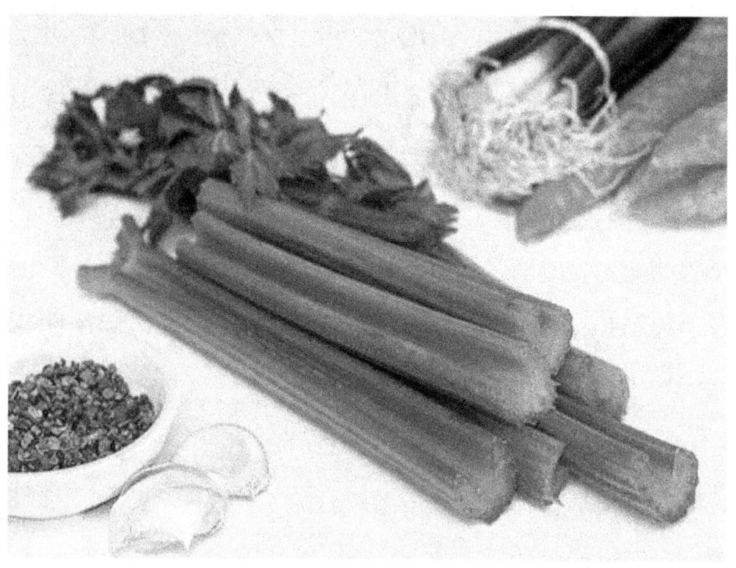

10. Carrots

Carrot is a favourite alkaline food for many people. It has all the different potential vitamins like A and C in it, in massive amounts that the body can then use with full zeal and glory. You can also choose to use them in the creation of your own fruit juices, such as the orange juice! You can also roast them in many different ways (some examples are rosemary roasted carrots, curry-spiced carrots, and spiced carrots) and they can serve as an excellent model of decoration for your barbecue. However, you must take care to not cook them too much, because a lot of cooking can make the food very acidic.

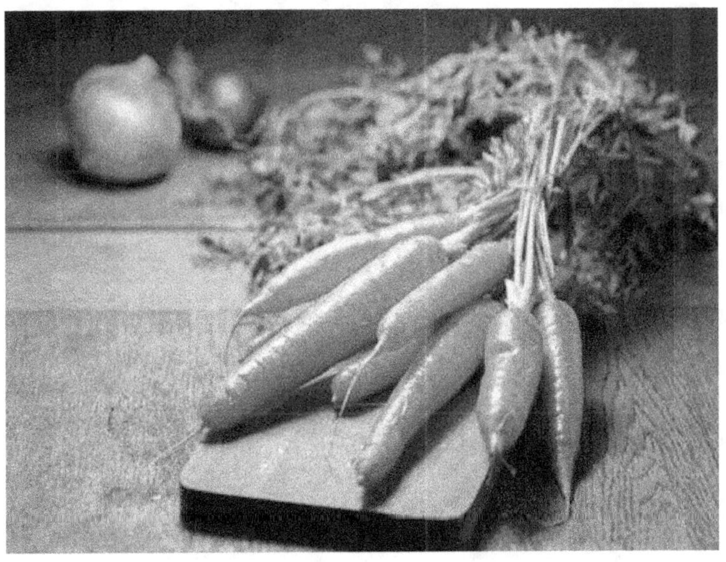

In addition, carrots contain antioxidants, which may protect against cancer and can help reduce the risks of cardiovascular disease. They are also rich in vitamins, minerals, and fiber.

11.   Sea Vegetables

Sea vegetables serve as excellent foods and supplements when you want to feed yourself with alkalinity. They are rich in magnesium, calcium, and sodium.

They are also embedded with vitamins like A, C and K, and hence they are typically eaten in a macrobiotic diet for this purpose.

Sea vegetables are also popular to have for their ocean-like flavour, and they make tasty additions to salads as well. Nori wraps are an excellent replacement to grain-based wraps.

12.   Sprouted Almonds

Almonds are an excellent choice for alkalizing, but they need to be used properly. For example, soaking and sprouting have many health benefits. They have many vitamins like E and C, and almonds are a great source of vegan protein and fibre. If you use sprouted almonds in a mixture, then they are sure to provide you with anti-inflammatory protection in no time.

13.   Bok Choy

This healthy food (cruciferous family of vegetables) is capable of transforming your body! Bok choy (or Chinese white cabbage) is packed with vitamins K and C and is very rich in antioxidants which helps to protect you against cancer. You can add bok choy to soups or salads, or you can even have it in wraps as well. In addition, bok choy contains folate, beta-carotene, and many important minerals like selenium, iron and zinc, that play crucial roles in the production and growth of collagen (very important for bone health). Some simple recipes containing Bok Choy are "sweet and spicy bok choy" and "Korean bok choy".

14. Raw Pumpkin Seeds

This beautiful supplement can be beneficial in improving your overall health regime. These seeds leave an alkaline ash in the blood when they are eaten, and thus they make the body more alkaline and purer.

They have a high amount of chlorophyll in their pigments, and because of this, the circulation of the human body becomes more agile and fast. They are also a great source of iron and protein, and they also make a sweet, crunchy addition to your desserts as well.

15. Pink Sea Salt

This Himalayan salt has a numerous amount of benefits for its consumers. This salt has over eighty-four per cent of minerals like magnesium, potassium, and calcium. As such, it can cure headaches, joint pain and fatigue, and even any muscle issues. If you know what to do with the salt, then you can easily buy and purchase it. You just need to consume it raw and then you can reap all the benefits of it!

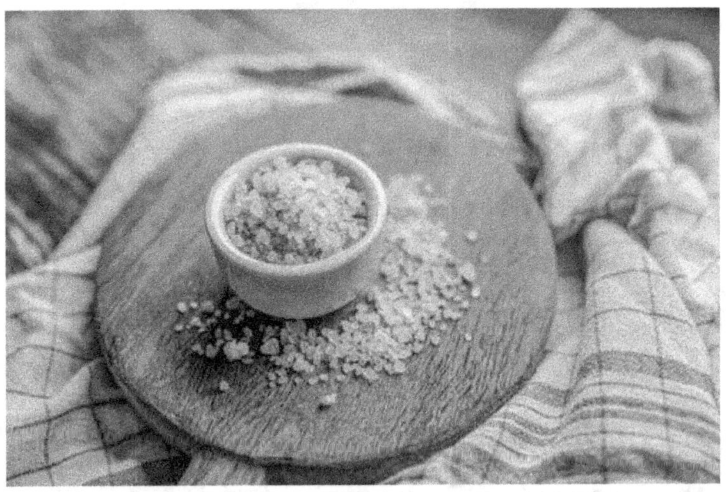

16. Matcha Green Tea

This green tea is not like regular green tea; instead, it has a considerable amount of nutrition for you. It is not heated or processed like any other tea, and it has an abundance of chlorophyll in it. Thus, It can improve your overall mood, and contains less caffeine and other acidic ingredients. It also has a considerable calming effect on your body, and if you want to start the day with a great amount of breakfast, then this Matcha Green Tea is sure to be the next big thing for you!

17. Spirulina

Do you want to have sea algae that will have a fantastic effect on the blood flow in your body? If you are searching for such, then spirulina is the next big thing for you. The nutrition of this food is very healthy; one tablespoon (or 7 grams) of dried spirulina contains four grams of protein, eight milligrams of calcium, 14 mg of magnesium, 95 mg of potassium, 2 mg of iron and other important elements.

Spirulina is a type of blue-green algae that people consider a superfood due to its excellent nutritional content and health benefits. It also contains thiamin, riboflavin, niacin, folate, phosphorous, and vitamins B-6, A, C and K.

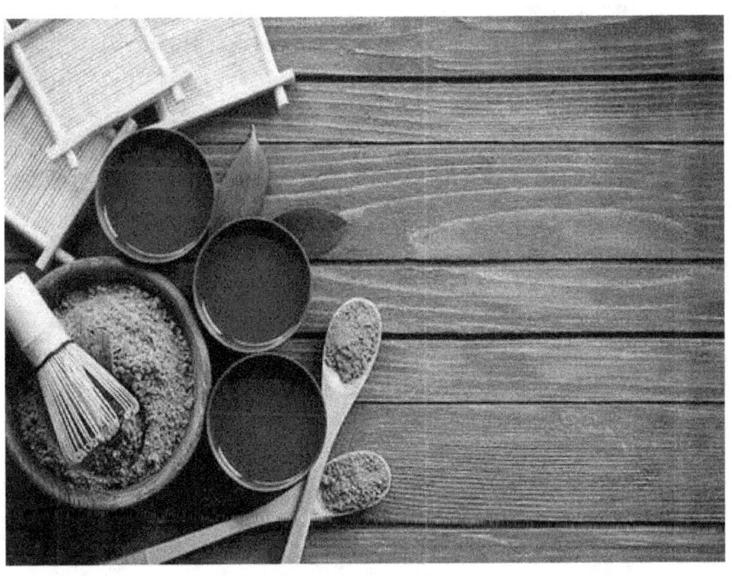

You can include spirulina in your diet in powder or tablet form. If you use it as a powder, you can add it to smoothies, on salads, in soups or into fruit or vegetable juices.

Thus, these are the alkalizing supplements that promote enriched healthy metabolic systems within our bodies and therefore promote good, strong, healthy growth. These supplements are all carefully examined, and they are easily attainable in a variety of different costs and packages.

CHAPTER 7

Breakfast recipes

If you want to start afresh in your daily routine, then you also must be able to choose fresh breakfast recipes for yourself. Breakfast is an essential part of any busy workday, and therefore, a breakfast must provide you with sufficient energy levels, and be packed full of nutrients and vitamins. An alkaline breakfast is fresh, packed with more nutrients than you could count, and can help you be productive in your day!

1.   French toast

This breakfast is widely shared and eaten throughout the world. French toast has all the necessary ingredients that boost energy within your body, and the ingredients are especially alkaline in their nature, thus promoting better health. French toast is also recommended by doctors to patients in order to help fight inflammatory diseases. This recipe is also easily made, by dipping pieces of bread into egg, and cooking. Then vanilla extract and cinnamon can bring a richness of flavor when making French toast.

The ingredients for this simple recipe are one egg, ¼ cup of milk, four slices bread, one teaspoon of vanilla extract and 1/2 teaspoon of ground cinnamon.

To prepare this tasty breakfast you have to beat egg, vanilla and cinnamon in a dish and then stir in milk. The next step is to dip bread in the mixture and then cook bread slices on the skillet on medium heat until browned on both sides. Now your French toast is finally ready to enjoy!

2.   Apple Pancakes

Apple pancakes are a great treasure for you if you strive for an alkaline diet, and with a cup of tea, apple pancakes are actually one of the healthiest alkaline meals of all. Whit this tasty and easy recipe you will find a beautiful mix of apples in the sweet aroma of cake batter!

To make them, you will need: 1½ cups of flour, 2 tablespoons of sugar (if you prefer you can use brown sugar), ¼ teaspoon of grounded cinnamon, 2 eggs (whisked), 2 teaspoons of baking powder, 1 teaspoon of baking soda, ½ teaspoon of salt, 1¼ cup of milk, two red apples (shredded), ¼ cup of applesauce, cooking oil (if necessary), blueberries and low-fat frozen yogurt. With these healthy ingredients, apple pancakes can be easily made.

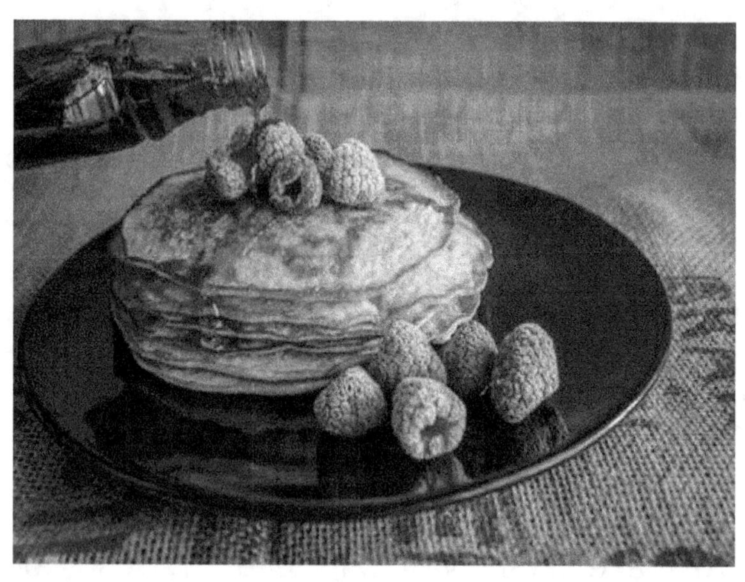

The instructions for preparing this breakfast are: in a large bowl, sift together flour, sugar (or brown sugar), baking powder, baking soda and salt. Whisk in milk, eggs, applesauce, and cinnamon just until combined; stir in shredded apples. Preheat a flat griddle over medium-high heat. Pour ¼ cup of pancake batter onto the griddle. Let pancakes cook until bubbles form before flipping.

Cook the other side until golden brown. Serve hot with syrup (for example maple syrup) and, if you want, you can add raspberries (or other fruit) and low-fat frozen yogurt.

3.   Avocado Breakfast Salad

This breakfast salad can help you regain all your lost energy when you are sleeping. It is the Mexican salad that can help give you the import micronutrients your body needs at all possible levels.

Its ingredients are a handful of corn tortilla chips (crumbled), half a spoon of firm tofu, one ripe avocado (peeled, pitted and sliced), one courgette (sliced), a handful of pumpkin seeds, a generous handful of chopped fresh cilantro, sea salt (if you prefer you can use Himalayan salt), ground pepper and half a lemon (fresh lemon juice).

It is incredibly simple to make, and perfect for anyone who wants a fast but extremely healthy diet!

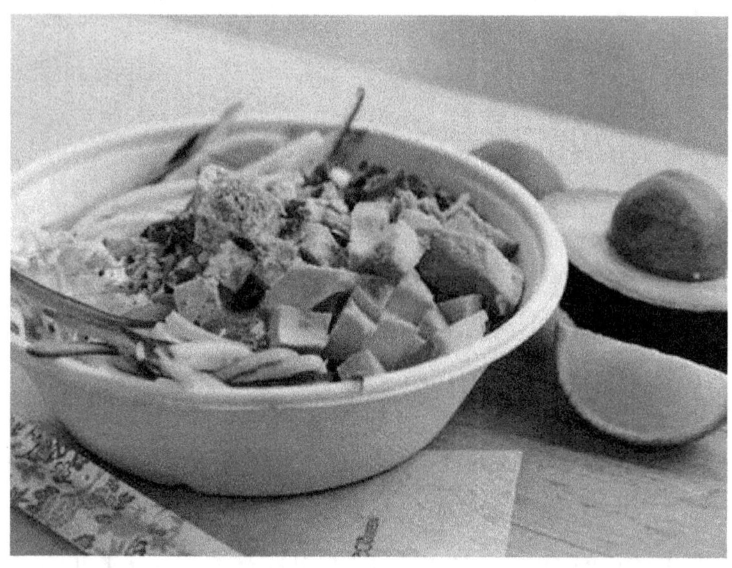

4.   Mixed Sprouts Salad

If you want to start your day with a tasteful alkaline diet then mixed sprouts is the best salad for you! It has umpteen amounts of proteins, vitamins, minerals and energy, which is extremely beneficial for you!

Its ingredients include one cup of sprouts, one cucumber (chopped), one red onion (chopped), a handful of parsley, fresh juice of a lemon, pink Himalayan salt, and ground black pepper. The making of it is also very simple (add all ingredients in a salad bowl, mix well and then garnish with fresh parsley), and it helps to give you the best amount of energy you can possibly achieve.

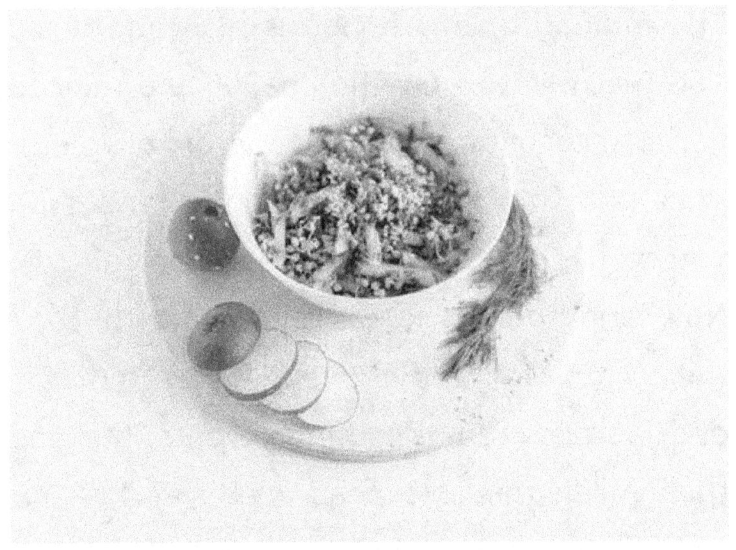

5.   Kale Chickpea Mash

This dish provides all the necessary benefits for you!

The ingredients are two tablespoons of garlic (minced), one shallot (minced), one bunch of kale, three hundred grams of fresh chickpeas, two tablespoons of coconut oil (or extra virgin olive oil) and Himalayan sea salt for more relish.

The making of this recipe is also effortless. You just need to fry the shallot and minced garlic in coconut oil (or extra virgin olive oil). Wait until it turns golden brown, and then you can add the kale (washed and drained). Now add the chickpeas and start to cook them, too (for about five minutes). In the end, add the remaining ingredients, stir and then mash the chickpeas with a fork. Your dish is finally ready to be served!

6.   Apple Cinnamon Quinoa Breakfast

This breakfast has healthy and delicious ingredients! These ingredients are ½ cup of uncooked quinoa (rinsed and drained), one cup of filtered water, one apple (peeled and diced), 1 teaspoon of ground cinnamon, ¼ teaspoon of ground ginger, and ½ cup of plain non-fat Greek yogurt (optional). These ingredients will produce the most excellent alkaline breakfast for you, because this meal has all the healthy proteins, enzymes and vitamins you need!

To create it, you have to cook the quinoa in a small saucepan (you have to add the cup of water; it is advised to boil the water for fifteen minutes or until the liquid is absorbed). Next, add the cinnamon, ginger and the diced apple, stir together and cook until the apples are tender (about 5 minutes). At the end of cooking, if you want, you can add two tablespoons of maple syrup, mixing well. Now your special breakfast is ready to be eaten!

7.   Cold Oats

This cold dish is a fantastic breakfast alkaline food for you that can give to your metabolism an amazing boost! The ingredients of this meal contain half a cup of oats, half a cup of milk (you can choose your favorite milk!), half a cup of yogurt, a pinch of salt, half a teaspoon of cinnamon, one banana (sliced), half a cup of berries and one tbsp of chia seeds (or other seeds, as you prefer!).

You can replace the banana and the berries with other fruit of your choice (like, for example, strawberries or raspberries). Instead, if you want a vegan recipe, you can choose nondairy yogurt and milk (options include almond, cashew, soy, rice, oat, or coconut).

The steps to preparing it are very simple to understand. Combine all ingredients in a jar, then shake well and refrigerate overnight. The next morning, simply stir, so it's absolutely delicious!

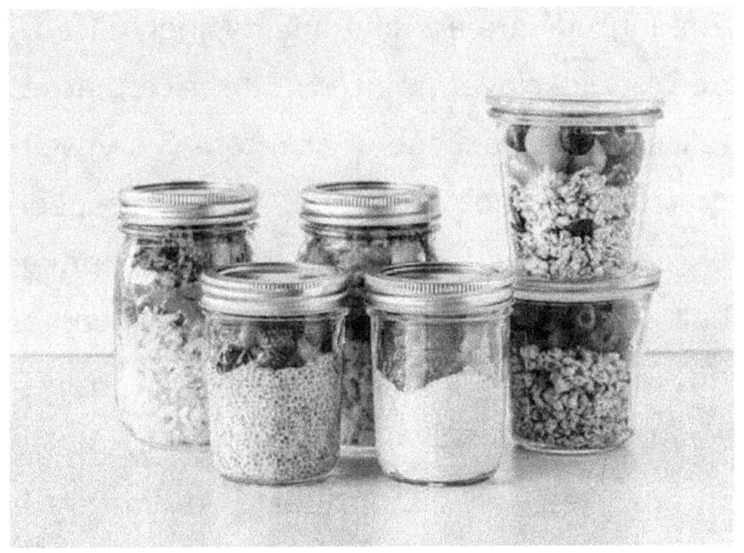

8.   Scrambled Tofu

Let's assume for one minute that you are a corporate business owner and you have to leave early for your job. For an extremely good lifestyle and great attention, the best possible breakfast that you can have is scrambled tofu! Its ingredients have a fantastic taste, and therefore, you can relish in all the energizing benefits but also still enjoy its consumption!

The ingredients are one onion (finely diced), one garlic clove (minced), three tomatoes (sliced), 1/2 package of firm tofu (very well-drained, but not pressed!), half a teaspoon of ground cumin, half a teaspoon of paprika, half a teaspoon of turmeric, one teaspoon of nutritional yeast, 2/3 cup of filtered water, 150g of baby spinach and a pinch of sea salt (or black salt, also known as "Kala Namak").

The steps to preparing this meal are: in a bowl combine turmeric, cumin, paprika, water, nutritional yeast and salt. Then add onion and garlic into a frying pan, and saute until fragrant (about 1-2 minutes). After doing this, crumble tofu into the pan (use your hands to break up the block of tofu) and pour the seasoning over tofu (it's necessary to mix well). Cook for 3 minutes or until tofu is hot throughout. Once cooked, add the tomatoes and the baby spinach, and this late addition will make the taste absolutely divine!

9.   Theplas

In the southern states of the Punjab region, Pakistan, and India, this recipe (theplas) is a Gujarati meal that is very alkaline in its creation.

The ingredients of this delicious recipe are: 1 teaspoon of coriander powder, 1 tablespoon of curd (yogurt), 1 teaspoon of red chilli powder, 1/2 teaspoon of turmeric powder, 1/2 cup of finely chopped spinach leaves (optional), 1/4 teaspoon of carom seeds (or sesame seeds), 1 cup + 1/2 cup of wheat flour, 2 teaspoons of oil (+ for shallow frying), salt and water.

These ingredients will create a perfect breakfast addition to your alkaline diet plan; however, some care is needed while preparing it!

The steps to prepare this dish are: first combine in a bowl one cup of wheat flour, spinach leaves, curd, red chilli powder, coriander powder, turmeric powder, 1 teaspoon of oil and salt. Next, add water as needed in small incremental quantities and knead a smooth and soft dough. After doing this, cover the dough with a plate and leave aside for 15-20 minutes. Then, divide it into seven equal parts. Now, take 1/2 cup of dry wheat flour in a plate for dusting. Take one dough ball, press it against the rolling board to flatten it and transform into a circle having approx. 6-7 inch diameter. Heat the griddle over medium flame and when it's hot, place raw thepla on it. When tiny bubbles appear on the top surface, flip it over and cook for 30 seconds. Flip it again, and cook the other side as well. Repeat the flip-cook process until light golden brown spots appear on both sides. Transfer it to a plate, then follow the same process for remaining dough balls. Gujarati theplas are now ready. Enjoy!

10. Maple Millet Porridge

The ingredients for this delicious breakfast, rich in proteins and amino acids, are one cup of millet, two cups of filtered water, one cup of unsweetened coconut milk, a pinch of salt, 1/4 tsp of cinnamon and maple syrup to taste. All these ingredients can be very prolific for the human body!

To prepare this fantastic alkaline breakfast, first, put the millet in a food processor and blend. Then add the processed millet in a saucepan with the milk, maple syrup, water, and cinnamon. Bring to the boil then turn the heat down to simmer and cook for around 15 minutes until it is very creamy. Serve in a bowl when it is ready and, if you want, top with fresh raspberries (100g) and pumpkin seeds (1 teaspoon).

It is highly encouraged to enjoy this breakfast often and incorporate it into your lifestyle, as not only is it delicious, but it is also incredibly easy to cook. You can have all the joy of eating great food, but also reap the benefits of maintaining an alkaline body state at the same time.

CHAPTER 8

Lunch Recipes

We have carefully examined and handpicked the best breakfast recipes for you, and now, it is time to discuss the best lunch recipes for you. Ideally, for an alkaline lunch recipe, we have fruits and other non-dairy products; however, many other lunch recipes can be used!

The lunch recipes are as follows:

1.   Summer Salad with citrus dressing

Do you have a busy lifestyle with not much time to prepare lunch? Salads make a fantastic, easy lunch and are extremely useful in maintaining an alkaline diet to improve health. To reap the best possible benefits, try to mix in a salad bowl ½ iceberg lettuce (shredded), two medium carrots (sliced), two large oranges (peeled and sectioned – you can use navel oranges), a handful of chia seeds, ¼ cup of chopped walnuts (optional), one tablespoon of extra virgin olive oil, ¼ cup of orange juice and two tablespoons of lemon juice. If you prefer a more salty taste, you can sprinkle some sea salt (if you prefer you can use pink Himalayan salt) on the salad for your own personal enjoyment!

This meal is beneficial in aiding in better health, and can be used in many situations where you want a quick lunch, but want the fantastic results that an alkaline diet can give you! By choosing this salad, you are sure to be getting all of those amazing results!

2.   Cheesy Kale Chips and Sliced Fruit

This recipe contains all the necessary amount of minerals, amino acids, proteins, and enzymes the human body needs! It's very simple to make and provide a lot of energy. This recipe also contains a sliced portion of fruit for you: fruit, coupled with these chips, can be very prolific for your health.

The ingredients for this tasty recipe are: 8 cups of kale and 2 cups of raw vegan cheese sauce (at the end you will find the recipe of this fantastic sauce).

The directions for preparing this lunch are: wash the kale and remove the stalks. Chop into bite-sized pieces. In a large bowl mix the raw vegan cheese sauce into the kale chips; make sure every inch of kale is coated with the sauce. Arrange the kale on a baking tray and bake for about 10 minutes at 300F/150C. Flip over the kale chips and bake for 10 minutes more. Keep a close eye on the kale chips as they burn easily. Store in an airtight container for up to 2 weeks. If the kale chips get soft, put them back in the oven for 5 minutes until crisp again. You can serve with a sliced portion of fruit.

Raw Vegan Cheese Sauce Recipe

You can prepare this tasty sauce with these ingredients: 1 cup of cashews, ½ cup of filtered water, 1 chopped red bell pepper, 2 tablespoons of lemon juice, ½ cup of nutritional yeast, 2 slices onion, 1 teaspoon of pink Himalayan sea salt (or sea salt), 1 teaspoon garlic powder and 2 teaspoons of onion powder.

The directions to prepare this sauce are: add all ingredients in a blender and blend for 60 seconds starting slow and increasing speed to high. Add water if needed.

3.   Green Apple Slices with Almond Butter

An almond contains infinite pieces of energy for your body, while apples are rich in fiber, Vitamin A, C, E, B-6, flavonoids, phytochemicals, potassium, calcium and iron.

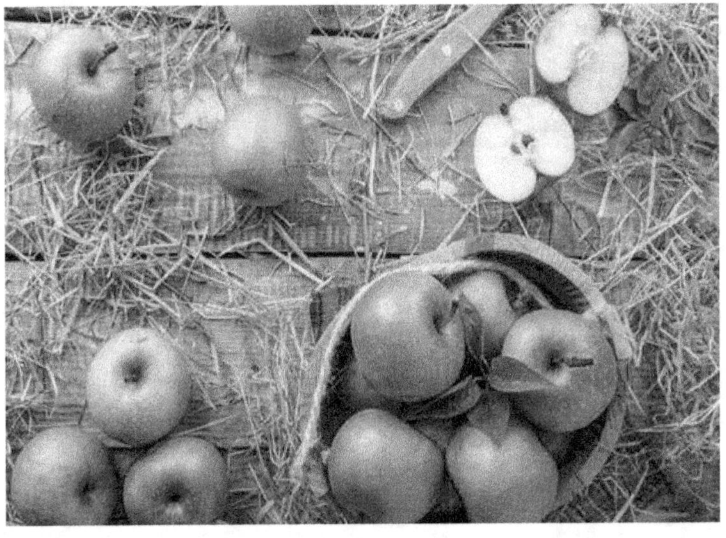

This recipe is very healthy and simple, because it has only these ingredients: one organic green apple, one scoop of almond butter (make sure no oil is added so you get more nutrients and less fat!) and organic honey (optional). Almond butter is a better choice than peanut butter, because almonds are rich in magnesium, vitamin E, iron, potassium, and calcium.

To prepare this dish you have to scoop some almond butter onto the middle of a plate and then place green apple slices around the almond butter. If you prefer, to sweeten the tartness of a green apple, you can add some honey on top.

4.   Apple, Red Cabbage & Beetroot Salad

This salad is very alkaline in its nature and can be helpful throughout the entire year! The ingredients to prepare this healthy recipe are one apple (cored and finely sliced), 500g of red cabbage (thinly sliced), 100g of raw beetroot (peeled and finely grated), 1 tbsp of cider vinegar, 2 tbsp extra-virgin olive oil,

30g of pomegranate seeds, fresh juice of a lemon, sea salt to taste (if you prefer you can use pink Himalayan sea salt) and small bunch parsley (chopped). The directions are very easy: combine all the ingredients in a large salad bowl and then serve!

5. Zucchini Sushi

The zucchini sushi will be just the lunch for you if you are a sushi lover and want to maintain an alkaline state to your body!

You can get all the enjoyment while making it, and your body will be able to perform well after eating it. The ingredients for this fabulous alkaline recipe are four zucchini (sliced), a quarter cup of parsley (minced), two artichoke hearts (cut in small pieces), two cloves of garlic (minced), one lemon (freshly juiced) and one can of white beans. You can slice the juicy zucchini in any way you choose, before mixing all the ingredients in a medium bowl for all possible tastes and flavours and maximum enjoyment!

6.   Courgette and Quinoa Salad

This recipe is very easy to prepare and the ingredients of this salad are very healthy for your body. They are: 300g of courgettes (washed and sliced), ½ cup of quinoa, 1 tsp of cumin, 400g of tin chickpeas (which are rinsed well and drained), 1 garlic clove (which is crushed with sea salt), 2 tablespoons of extra virgin olive oil, 2 tablespoons of lemon juice, 2 spring onions (chopped), and a small handful of flat-leaf parsley leaves (chopped).

The directions to create this tasty recipe are really simple. Add the quinoa to a pot, then add a cup of water, and bring to the boil over medium heat before simmering it for ten minutes or until all the water is absorbed.

Replace the lid and prepare all the other ingredients. After doing it, heat the extra virgin olive oil in a large pan. Addition of the courgettes is the next step. While cooking, stir until bright green and tender. Spoon into a bowl, season and then set aside. Replace the pan over medium heat; add the cumin and cook, stirring until fragrant. In the last step, add the chickpeas, quinoa, garlic, lemon juice, spring onions, and parsley and toss well. Now, you're ready to serve!

7.   Cauliflower Gnocchi

This dish is vegan and excellent in its creation and it will yield you fantastic results for your health!

The ingredients include one head of cauliflower (steamed or boiled), one garlic clove (chopped), one cup of flour, one tablespoon of olive or coconut oil to fry.

Instead, for the ragout, you need one tin of whole tomatoes, four courgettes (sliced), half an onion (finely sliced), one tablespoon of olive or coconut oil, one garlic clove (chopped), five large black mushrooms (sliced), three hundred milliliters of vegetable stock and one tsp of sugar. In the end, salt to taste and fresh basil to serve.

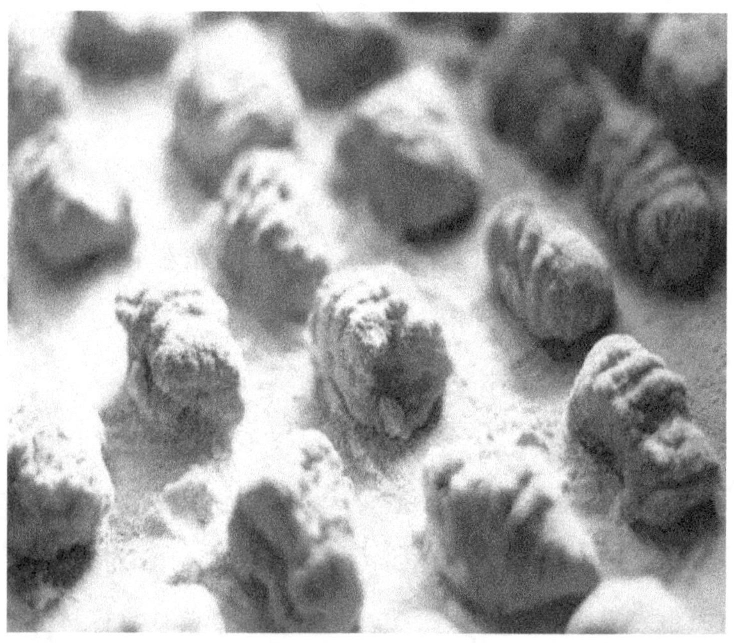

The directions to prepare this delicious recipe are: place the cauliflower and garlic in a blender (or food processor) and blend until smooth. Then, add a little water (if needed), salt and flour (1/4 cup at a time) and continue to process until a soft dough is formed. Turn out on a floured surface and knead briefly until dough is soft. Cut dough into four pieces, take one and roll out into a rope approximately 3 cm, then cut into 3cm pieces (after doing it, repeat with remaining dough). Now you're ready for cooking: place the olive oil (or coconut oil) in a non-stick pan and fry the gnocchi until lightly browned on both sides.

Instead, for the ragout, place the olive oil (or coconut oil) in a non-stick pot over medium-high heat. Add the onion, garlic, mushrooms and courgettes and fry until starting to colour and soften. Add the tomatoes, vegetable stock and sugar, reduce to medium heat and allow to gently simmer for 20 minutes - until the vegetables are tender. Serve the ragout with the warm cauliflower gnocchi on top and then scattered with basil leaves. Now you are ready to enjoy it!

8.   Kale and Cucumber Kimchi

Kimchi is a popular Korean side dish, packed with beneficial nutrients. In short words, kimchi is a fermented vegetable dish that gives you a great amount of protein, amino acids and triggers pro-active digestion in your body. This dish can help you with conditions like inflammation and digestive issues.

The ingredients of this particular recipe are 250g of white cabbage (sliced), 250g of kale (chopped), 250g of cucumber (diced), sea salt, 2 tbsp. of dried chili flakes, 1 tbsp. of smoked paprika, 3 garlic cloves (minced), 1 tbsp. of fresh ginger (finely grated) and 500ml of mineral water.

The directions to prepare this healthy recipe are: combine the cabbage, kale, cucumber and salt together, then squeeze the vegetables, with your hands, for five minutes. With this method, natural water can easily come out of the vegetables and will provide a great amount of taste. After doing this, stir in the rest of the ingredients and transfer it to a sterilized jar with a lid.

Tips: leave it on the kitchen counter, away from direct sunlight, and fermentation of the mixture will take place (the recommended time is three weeks before tasting). Transfer it to the fridge once you are ready with the taste.

9.   Cauliflower Tabbouleh Salad

This salad is very alkaline and thus is extremely beneficial for your health and for your body energy!

The ingredients to prepare this tasty recipe are one raw head of cauliflower (coarsely chopped), two onions (chopped), 2 cups (packed) of flat-leaf parsley leaves with tender stems (minced), 1 cup (packed) of mint leaves (minced), ½ cucumber (finely diced), 150g of cherry tomatoes (quartered), 1 garlic clove (coarsely chopped), 1/4 teaspoon of crushed red pepper flakes, 3 tablespoons of extra-virgin olive oil, and sea salt to taste. In the end, the juice of one small lemon will add that little bit more flavour!

The method is very crucial, as, in a tabbouleh salad, the cauliflower must be dried, washed and cut correctly. Cut the cauliflower into chunks and add it into a food processor. Any process of cutting it down is ok, but it needs to be extremely fine in its consistency. Now, for cooking the cauliflower, heat the pan over medium heat. Add a bit of extra virgin olive oil, and cook the cauliflower until brown (continue heating and stirring until cauliflower starts to release some of its moisture and is crisp-tender). When cauliflower is cool, place in a large salad bowl with cucumber, tomatoes, onions, garlic, red pepper flakes, extra virgin olive oil, sea salt, mint and parsley. Then, add the lemon juice for a fresh and authentic taste!

10. Grilled Courgette Salad

The best alkaline dish that you can taste for maintaining a healthy body is a grilled courgette salad! There are spicy ingredients too that can slightly boost metabolism, increasing the number of calories you burn throughout the day.

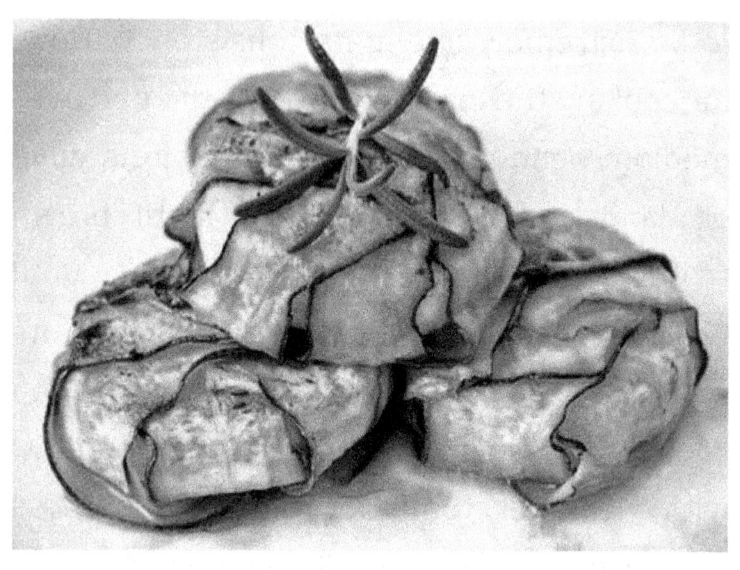

The ingredients to prepare this easy recipe are 6 courgettes, 1 red chilli, a handful of fresh mint leaves, extra virgin olive oil, freshly ground black pepper and sea salt (if you prefer you can use pink Himalayan sea salt).

To prepare this fantastic meal, slice the courgettes lengthwise (as thin as you can) and then grill on a griddle pan (or on the barbecue), until lightly charred on each side. Scatter the slices over a large plate and then sprinkle them with a little sea salt and freshly ground black pepper. Now, wash the mint leaves and red chilli and chop finely, then sprinkle the chilli and mint evenly from a height over the courgettes. To finish, drizzle with good extra virgin olive oil.

All these ingredients will create an intense flavour experience for you to enjoy!

11.   Roasted Vegetable and Coconut Milk soup

This dish is very alkaline and beneficial for you!

The ingredients of this lunch include 2 cups of mixed vegetables (chopped into chunks), 20ml of extra virgin olive oil (which is used to roast vegetables), sea salt and black pepper to taste, 1 tablespoon of coconut oil, 2 cloves garlic (peeled and crushed), 1 tin of coconut milk and a bit of freshly grated ginger.

First and foremost, arrange the chopped vegetables in an oven-safe baking tray (drizzle with extra virgin olive oil). Then, roast in the oven at 180 degrees Celsius until soft (about 30 minutes). In the meantime, in a saucepan, heat the coconut oil and saute the garlic and ginger for a few minutes. Now, add the coconut milk and simmer for 20 minutes on medium-low heat, until reduced by a quarter. When the milk is ready, transfer it to a soup bowl and then add the roasted vegetable. Serve hot!

12.   Crunchy quinoa salad

This salad is perfect and delicious and it is great for your healthy state of mind. The ingredients contain 1 cup of uncooked quinoa, 1 1/2 cups of fresh cauliflower (chopped in pieces), extra virgin olive oil, 1 cucumber (sliced), 1 raw carrot (sliced), ½ cup of kale, 1 teaspoon of chopped fresh mint, 2 tablespoons of chopped fresh parsley, 3 tablespoons of lemon juice, a pinch of pumpkin seeds, sea salt (if you prefer you can use pink Himalayan sea salt) and freshly ground black pepper.

The directions of this delicious recipe are: rinse the quinoa well and place it in a pot with water and bring to a boil. Cover and cook for 15 minutes. Remove from the heat, stir, and allow the quinoa to cool slightly.

Meanwhile, put a large pot of water on the stove to boil, drop the cauliflower and kale into the boiling water, and cook for 5 minutes, until crisp-tender (above all the cauliflower). Remove from the pot with a slotted spoon and drop into a bowl. Then drain. After doing this, combine the cooked quinoa, cauliflower, cucumber, carrot, and kale in a salad bowl. Add the remaining ingredients and mix well. Season with freshly ground black pepper and sea salt (if desired).

CHAPTER 9

Dinner Recipes

We all want a satisfying and delicious dinner to end our daily routines, but we also want a dinner that gives us less fat while we are sleeping! To satisfy these needs, we have to search and come up with meals that are high in alkalinity. These are the dinners which make your bodies look lean and fit, and aesthetic. Moreover, they will improve your overall health and wellbeing (below are some recipes for some fantastic alkaline dinners).

1.   Beetroot Latte

Beetroot latte can be very helpful for your body as it provides an enormous amount of energy! If you also add one cup of almond milk in the latte, it will be beneficial for you. The beetroot latte is also very colourful, and it is lovely and creamy. It combines all the best ingredients and even helps regulate blood pressure; this recipe is very easy to prepare!

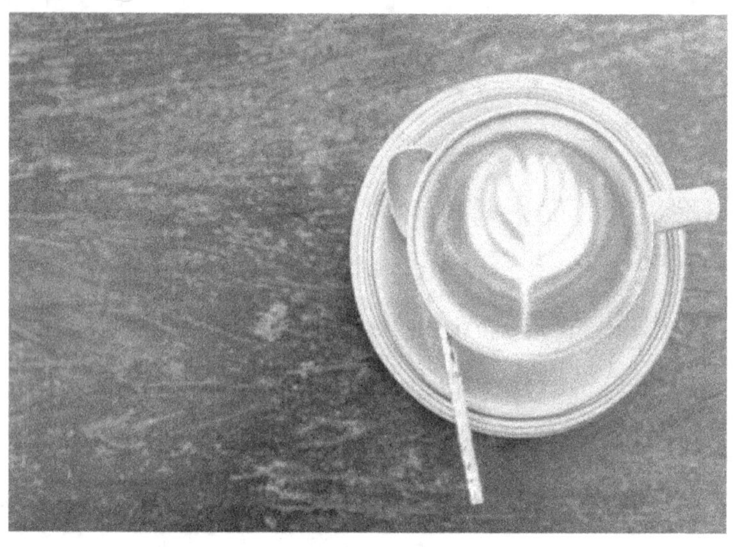

The ingredients to prepare beetroot latte are: one shot of fresh beetroot juice (or two teaspoons of beet powder), one teaspoon of honey (it's important to use a good quality of honey, better if it's organic!), one cup of unsweetened almond milk, and a sprinkle of cinnamon (this ingredient is optional). Now warm the milk and the honey in a saucepan (do not boil!). Then, if you prefer, froth the milk.

The next step is to combine one shot of beetroot juice (or two teaspoons of beet powder), with the frothed milk and then to sprinkle with a dash of cinnamon (if desired). However, do ensure you mix the ingredients well.

2.   Gluten-Free Berry & Red Currant Pie

To prepare this fantastic recipe, the ingredients are one prepared unbaked pie crust (gluten-free), fresh fruit (for example you can use 500g of red currant and 500g of blueberries), ¼ cup of sweetener of your choice (you can use organic honey), zest and juice from half a lemon, 3 tablespoons of cornstarch, ½ cup of oats, ½ cup white rice flour, 2 tablespoons of brown sugar and 4 tablespoons of butter (melted and cooled slightly).

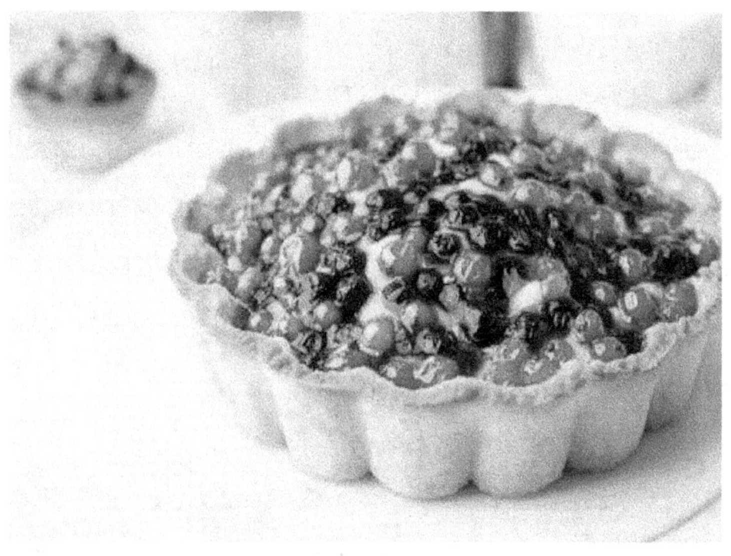

To prepare the pie filling, you have to combine the rice flour, oats, brown sugar and melted butter in a small bowl. Then, place in the fridge (about 30 minutes). After doing this, preheat the oven to 180 degrees Celsius.

The next step is to prepare the fruit (topping): in a large bowl, combine blueberries, red currant, honey, lemon zest, lemon juice, and cornstarch and toss until they are well combined. Then pour the pie filling into the pie crust. Cover with the fruit topping. Bake in preheated oven approximately 60 minutes, until pie crust is golden brown. Let cool completely before serving (you can place it in the fridge to finish cooling).

3.   Spicy Cashews

A beautiful and rich dish is what you will find in the spicy cashews. This recipe is very easy and flavorful, especially good the next day. It is an absolutely fantastic meal to serve at dinner time and it is recommended by families far and wide, receiving a great deal of affection when it is served on the dinner table!

The ingredients of this recipe are two cups of raw cashews, two tablespoons of butter, one tablespoon of canola oil, 1 teaspoon of sea salt, ½ teaspoon of chili powder and ¼ to ½ teaspoon of crushed red pepper flakes.

In a large frying pan, saute cashews in oil and butter for 5 minutes, stirring continuously, until golden brown. Spread on a paper towel-lined baking sheet; let stand for 3 minutes. Transfer to a wide bowl and sprinkle with pepper, salt and chili powder, then toss well. Store the cashews in an airtight container once they cool to room temperature (they can be stored up to a month).

There are many bursting flavours within this recipe, but better yet, it is helping to maintain alkaline levels in your body too. The dish is inspired by the Indian recipes like the potato and cauliflower curry, the spicy aloo gobi, okra masala, and even the banana cardamom lassi. These are all recipes that can be used in many different ways to keep your body in a state of alkalinity while you sleep.

CHAPTER 10

Dessert Recipes

Dessert is, of course, an important part for every individual after any meal! It gives a sweet enjoyment and it is very effective for your health gives even more satisfaction to you once you are done eating your food. The dessert recipes that can give a sweet alkaline taste to you are as follows:

1.   Vanilla Coconut Chia Pudding

A very easy and delicious alkaline recipe for you: the vanilla coconut chia pudding.

Ingredients:

- two cups of coconuts
- half a cup of raw cashews
- two tablespoons coconut oil
- a quarter of a teaspoon of salt

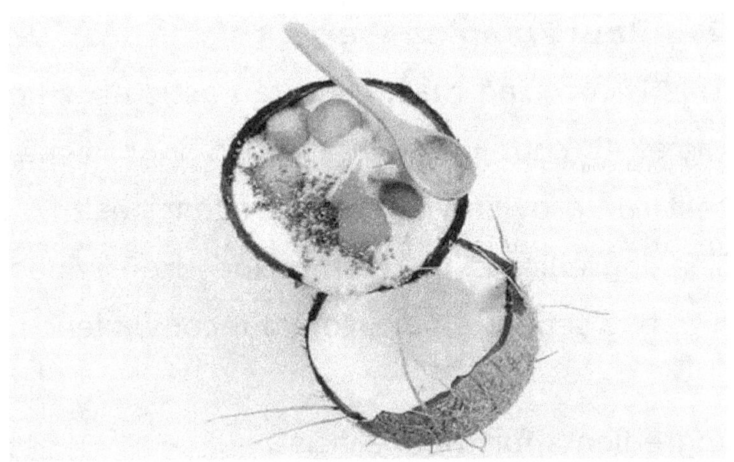

Its preparation directions are also very important, as you must ensure it is stirred properly. Except for the chia and pomegranate seeds, put the mixture in a blender and blend them thoroughly. Variety can also be included in this recipe, and you could add a quarter of a cup of raw cacao before the first blend.

2.   Raw Pumpkin Pie

This is a recipe that has a fantastic alkaline taste! It contains all the fresh ingredients that can provide you with excellent health. The ingredients for this recipe are divided into two separate parts for your convenience.

Ingredients for the pie crust:
- a cup of raw almonds
- one cup of unsweetened coconut flakes
- one cup of dates and Turkish apricots
- and one teaspoon of cinnamon

Ingredients for the pie filling:
- one cup of pecans
- one cup of organic pumpkin puree
- six dates
- half a teaspoon of cinnamon
- half a teaspoon of nutmeg
- a quarter of sea salt
- one teaspoon of gluten-free tamari

The method used for creating both the pie filling and the pie crust is different, and thus you must take care to ensure you are following the correct one!

Blend the pie crust ingredients until the oils come out of the mixture. Then you have to place it in a mould, or, if you prefer, you could also use a pie pan for it. After putting it in the mould, push it around gently until it covers the whole of the mould.

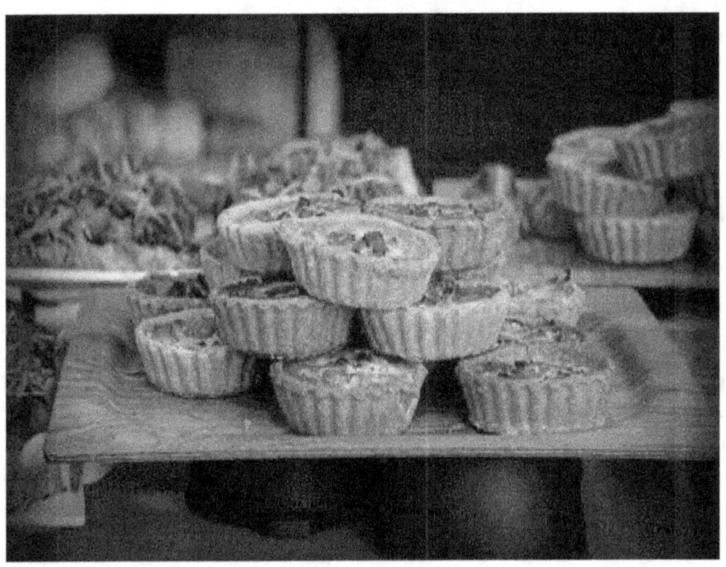

For the pie filling, you have to blend the ingredients well. Then, once done, add the mixture into the pie crust, and you at this point, you can also sprinkle cinnamon on top of it for extra taste!

3.   Frozen Chocolate Tropical Monkey

If you had a hot day and you want to have a frozen chocolate tropical monkey, then it could actually be extremely beneficial for your health as well! There are many characteristics to a frozen chocolate tropical monkey. It is sweet, delicious, filled with flavour, and it has many interesting alkaline properties to it. There is also no need to add acidic ice-cream into it to give it better flavour, simply because it already has an alkaline taste!

Ingredients:

- two frozen bananas
- two tbsp. coconut oil
- two tbsp. cocoa powder
- two tbsp. cocoa nibs
- two tbsp. chia seeds
- two cups of coconut milk

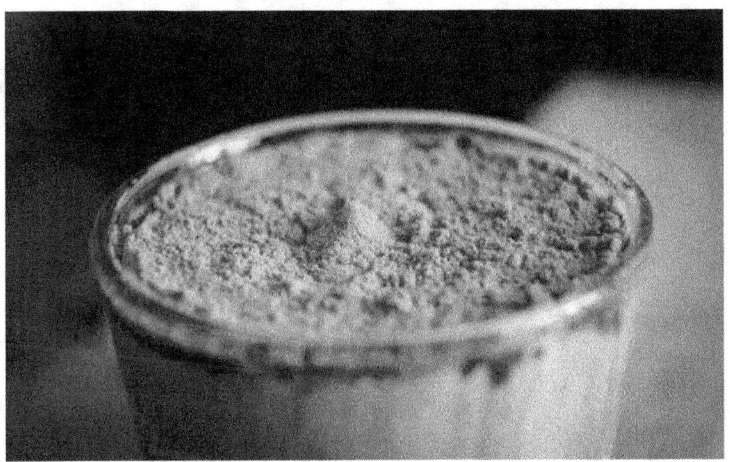

The directions for preparing it are incredibly simple! First, you need to mix all the ingredients in the mixer and then add the chia seeds to give more taste to it. In this way, you have the sweetest alkaline dessert you could ever possibly imagine.

4.   Dairy-Free Berry Parfaits

This recipe is just right for an easy summer dessert and it is just the thing that a bodybuilder or any corporate worker needs these days. You have to add berries to it, which create a great deal of flavour, and by following this regime, gives it that proper taste. You just have to be active while you are baking it.

Ingredients:

- 5 gluten-free graham crackers
- 2 tablespoons vegan buttery spread
- 5 ounces Coco Whip (coconut whipped topping made with organic coconut oil)
- 1/2 cup strawberries chopped
- 1/2 cup blackberries

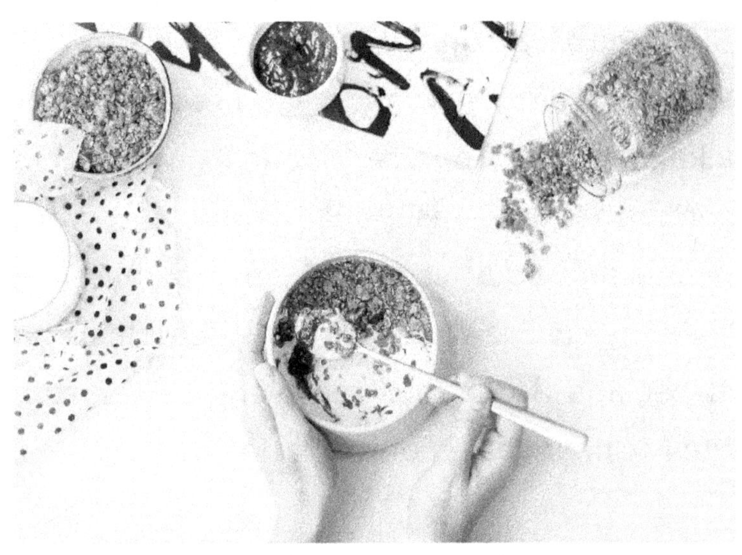

Place the crackers in a food processor, until they become fine crumbs. Add the vegan buttery spread and process until the mixture comes together. Spoon some of the graham cracker crust mixture into the bottom of six small jars and add some Coco Whip and some berries. Then repeat, until you fill each jar. Serve immediately.

5.   Healthy Collard Wraps

Want a healthy fast and vegan recipe that is alkaline in nature, and will give comprehensive results to improving your health and body shape? Then you must try "healthy collard wraps"! This vegetable has a sweet and a delicious taste and better still, the recipe involves only a little cooking.

The recipe is completely packed with vegetables and the nutrient content is really strong. But, at the same time, this dish is low in calories. The collards are one of those greens that are packed with good-for-you nutrients. The health benefits of collards include protein, fiber, chlorophyll and tons of other vitamins.

The ingredients of this recipe are: collard (4 leaves), hummus (1/2 cup), cooked quinoa (1 cup), one cucumber, one tomato, two grated carrots, one sliced avocado and sprouts (1/2 cup).

Instructions: cook the leaves in boiling water for 15-20 seconds. Then spread the hummus into the center of each leaf, then top with quinoa, cucumber, tomato, grated carrots, sliced avocado and finishing with the sprouts. In the end, fold in the sides, take the edge facing you and fold it over the ingredients.

6.   Mediterranean kale salad with Golden Raisins

This salad is very special for its consumer. This raw food diet, which might sound a little drastic and scary, can be highly effective for the body as it contains vitamins, enzymes and other nutritional compositions as well. To prepare this delicious meal, you just need Mediterranean salads and leaves and they must be covered with golden raisins to give an extra flavor boost! You will also need to de-stem your kale. It is also recommended that you check out Leah Putnam's premium videos on Grokker, which is an online platform promoting health and wellbeing.

7.   Easy Tropical Fruit Tart

If you are fond of French dishes but you also want to maintain an alkaline state, then you must follow and try out the recipe for this dessert! It is an easy tropical fruit tart.

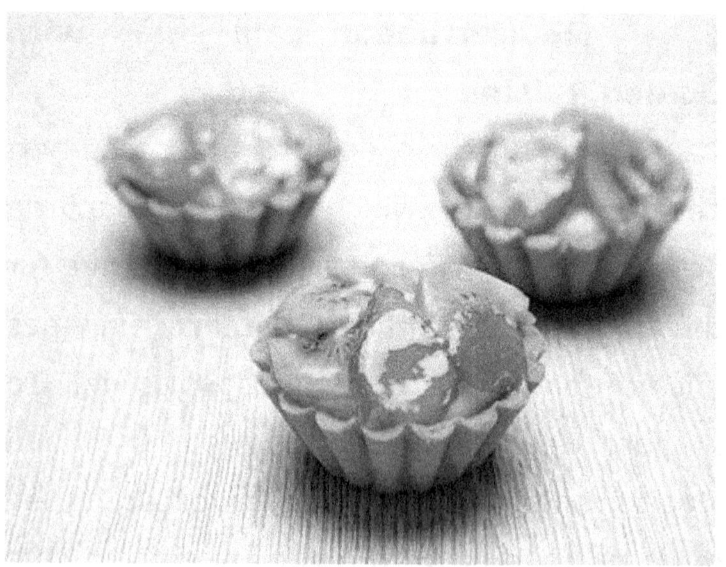

Having fruits on it gives you a multitude of minerals, vitamins and healthy enzymes. It has the flavors of coconut, macadamia, Medjool, mangoes, kiwi, and strawberries. It, therefore, allows you to maintain the strong PH of your body while eating it and enjoying its incredible taste, but also allows you to reap the enormous health benefits it provides in no time!

For a quick recipe, you can buy packaged little tarts (ready to use), and you can do the same with the pastry cream (you can buy packaged pastry cream ready to use). Then, you can use only kiwi and strawberries on the pastry cream (in a few words take the tart, fill it with the pastry cream and then add kiwi and strawberries on top).

8.   Peanut Butter Ice Cream

Ingredients:

*   ¾ cup smooth peanut butter

*   2/3 cup sugar

*   3 cups half-and-half (a combo of half

milk and half cream)

*   1 teaspoon vanilla

*   1/8 teaspoon salt

*   a cup of spring water

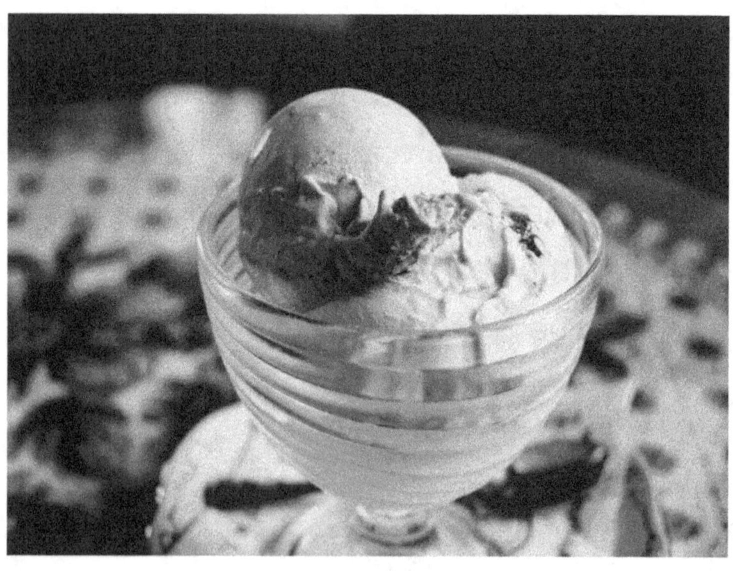

The directions to create this recipe must be understood fully to get the required result. Beat peanut butter and sugar until smooth. Slowly beat in one cup half and half until thoroughly combined. Whisk in two cups half and half, vanilla and salt. Freeze the liquid mixture for 30 minutes and then mix until you get a smooth and creamy consistency, which is just right for the dessert.

9. Kale smoothie

Smoothie made with kale? Yes, it's true, and it's truly delicious, too! This smoothie, tastes like ice cream, is the most incredible green smoothie you will ever taste.

Ingredients:

*   1 cup of torn-up curly green kale leaves
*   ¼ cup of chopped pitted dates
*   1/2 cup of raw unsalted cashews, soaked

- 2 bananas

- 1/2 teaspoon natural vanilla extract

- 1 teaspoon minced ginger

- 1 cup of filtered water

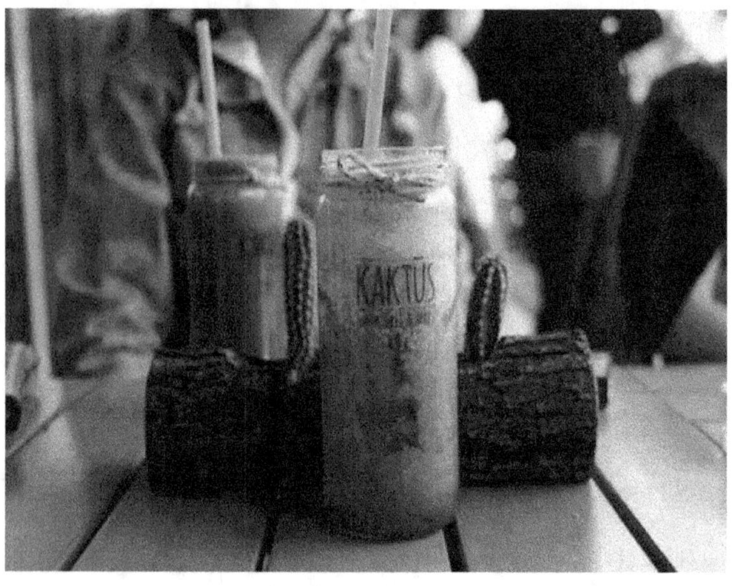

Place the chopped pitted dates in a little bowl. Cover them with filtered water and allow to sit for about 15 minutes to soften. Pour the water and dates into the blender, add the other ingredients and blast on high for 30 seconds (or more), until smooth and creamy.

Following these instructions, you will have the perfect, most delicious kale smoothie in no time!

The recipes have been essential alkaline dessert recipes that you must try before and after any lunch intake! The idea is a straightforward one, and it is recommended that you share it with all of your friends! You will soon see yourself looking better in the mirror and thank yourself for starting this diet, and whether it is breakfast, lunch, or even a dessert, you will soon see that the alkalinity of your body matters a lot!

CHAPTER 11

Fantastic smoothie and other easy recipes

This chapter contains smoothie and other easy recipes that are not only tasty but are perfect for an alkaline diet. They are simple, easy to make, and have terrific health benefits! They are as follows:

Avocado Lime Smoothie

The avocado lime smoothie is the real deal! Both avocados and limes are easily available and even better; the avocado contains minerals, vitamins and enzymes, which are extremely beneficial. This recipe is great for weight loss, vision, osteoporosis prevention, and is good for cancer-fighting.

Ingredients:

- 75g cucumber with the peel
- 85g baby spinach
- 200g frozen broccoli
- 75g avocado
- 115g organic silken tofu
- two small limes, peeled
- half teaspoon of stevia
- half a cup of ice
- half a cup of unsweetened organic plant-based milk

To prepare, add all the ingredients together into a high-speed blender and blend it all together, then serve to all the people you want to share with!

SuperSpeed Spelt Pancakes

Ingredients:

* ¼ cup of pumpkin seeds

* ¼ cup of sesame seeds

* ¼ cup of flax seeds

* ¼ cup of chia seeds

* 1 cup of buckwheat groats (or spelt flour)

* half teaspoon of baking powder

* one teaspoon of baking soda

* half teaspoon of sea salt

* two teaspoons of plant-based milk

* one teaspoon of coconut oil

* half teaspoon of stevia

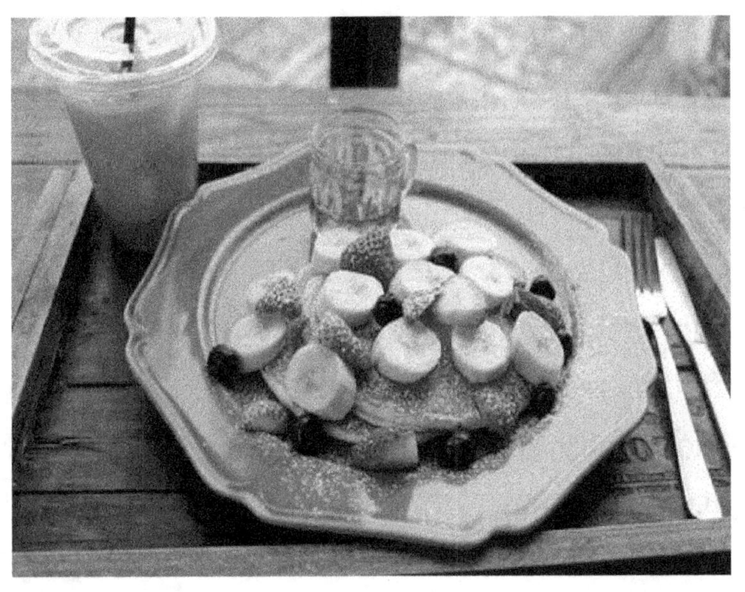

First and foremost, you need to grind the first five ingredients into the flour. Then, store a quarter of the seed flour next and set aside. Combine two cups of your seed flour in a medium bowl. Add the remaining ingredients except for the coconut oil, and add more milk until it reaches the right consistency. You need to preheat the non-stick pan with coconut oil, pour thin layers of pancakes and flip once bubble appears on top. You have to continue this step until your mixture is finished. This diet is very nutritional for you, and you must come up with a healthy appetite for it if you wish to carry this diet forward!

This recipe is excellent for weight loss, cardiovascular disease, lowering high cholesterol, preventing diabetes, managing diabetes, digestion, for detox purposes and fighting heart disease.

Healing and Nourishing Vegetable Soup

This is a tasty and healing alkaline soup for you to enjoy that can be easily eaten in any situation. The healing and nourishing vegetable soup will soon be the first thing that will come to your mind when you think of fast and healthy smoothies!

Ingredients:

- 1 large onion, diced
- 3 celery (full-length stick)
- 3 carrots
- 3 garlic cloves, minced
- 1/2 cup of fresh parsley
- 1 tsp fresh rosemary, de-stemmed and chopped
- 1 yeast-free vegetable stock powder
- 2 cups of chopped cauliflower
- 3 cups of chopped green beans
- 1/2 teaspoon sea salt
- a pinch of ground pepper
- two liters of pure water

To prepare this soup, you have to chop all the ingredients, and then you must cook them for thirty minutes, before serving in a bowl of long grain basmati rice. This recipe is excellent for you in terms of weight loss, cancer-fighting, detoxing, feeling less stressed, anti-inflammatory, preventing heart disease, lowering blood pressure, diabetes and preventing grout.

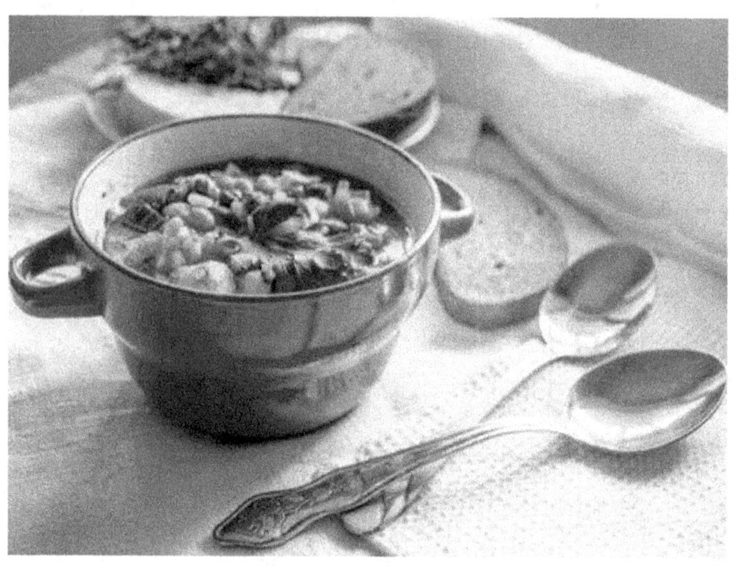

Warming Blueberry Porridge

If you are a beginner in the world of alkaline dieting, then this warming blueberry porridge is great!

Ingredients:

- ¼ cup of buckwheat groats
- 1 tablespoon of chia seeds
- 10 almonds
- 1/2 cup of unsweetened almond milk
- ¼ teaspoon of ground cinnamon
- a pinch of stevia and blueberries

To prepare, you will need to soak the buckwheat groats with pure water overnight. You will need to soak the chia seeds and almonds, and you will need to drain the buckwheat and also rinse it well. Then, you will need to add the buckwheat and unsweetened almond milk to a nonstick pan and cook for seven minutes. Once you have cooked it, then you may serve it in a bowl and to top it off with the yummy fresh berries! It will have a delicious taste, which will be very helpful for the beginners.

The recipe is essential for good heart health; it can also lower high cholesterol, reduces hypertension and it is good for digestion. This dish relieves constipation and lowers high blood pressure; it is gluten-free, it fights depression, anxiety and also prevents severe headaches.

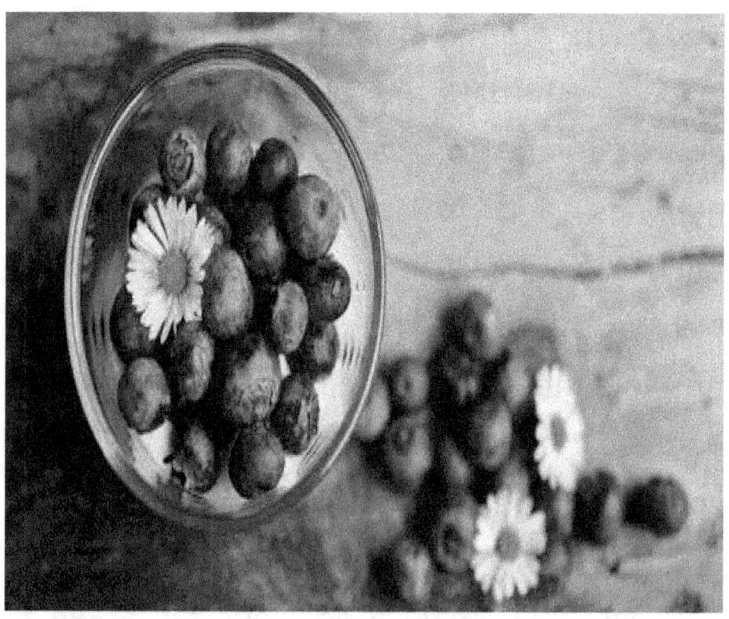

Unrivaled Chocolate Chia Pudding

If you are a chocolate lover, but you also want to maintain an alkaline state to your body, then this Unrivaled Chocolate Chia pudding is the absolute best dessert for you!

Ingredients:
- ¼ cup of chia seeds
- 1 teaspoon of vanilla extract
- 1 heaped teaspoon of 100% cocoa powder
- a pinch of ground cinnamon
- 2 cups unsweetened almond milk (or your favorite non-dairy milk)

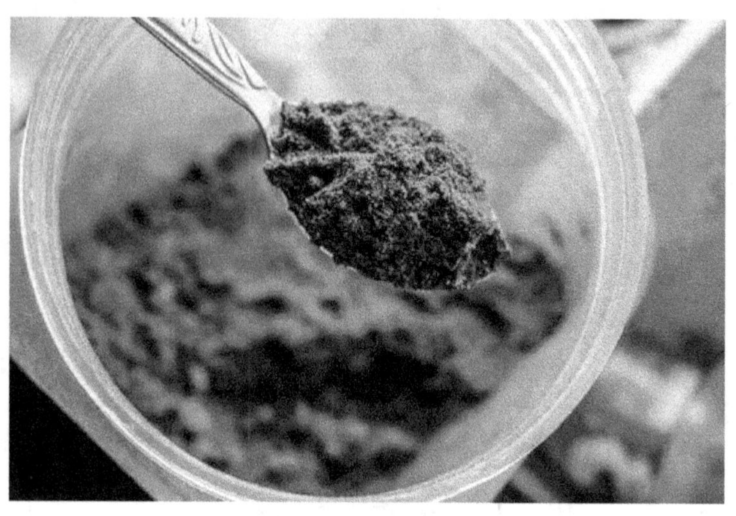

To create this fabulous chocolate pudding, combine all of the ingredients in a mixing bowl and mix them really well. Place the mix into a jar and store overnight, stirring it well before serving the next morning.

The recipe is great for weight loss, it treats diverticulosis, it helps cardiovascular disease, it lowers high cholesterol, it prevents and manages diabetes, it is great for digestion, it helps forms of detox and it fights heart disease.

Lean Green Fennel Smoothie

The ingredients for this tasty alkaline smoothie are:

- 135g cucumber
- two cups of spinach
- half a fennel bulb
- a quarter of a cup of fresh mint leaves
- two servings of avocado
- one teaspoon of chia seeds
- one serving of sprouted rice

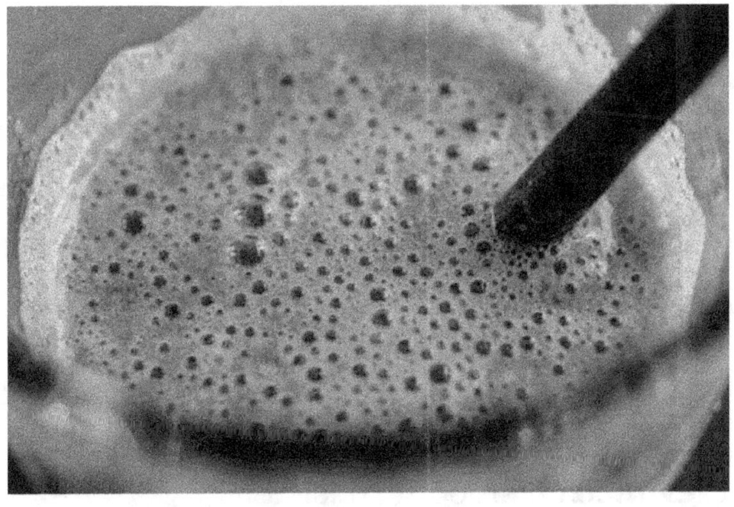

Directions:

Add all the ingredients together into a powerful high-speed blender, and blend until you get a consistency that is smooth and creamy for ultimate enjoyment!

Alkalizing Super Shake

Ingredients:

- one cucumber
- two kale leaves
- 30g fresh ginger
- two serves of avocado
- one cup of fresh coconut water
- one tablespoon of fresh mint
- juice of one lime
- ¼ cup of chia seeds

Add all of the ingredients into a powerful high-speed blender and blend them until they reach a smooth consistency.

This smoothie contains all the health benefits needed for maintaining alkalinity for your body.

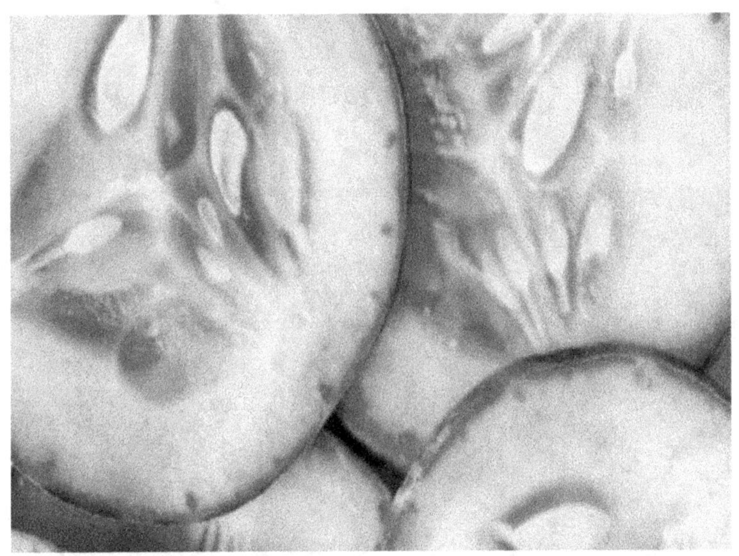

Coconut-Lime Smoothie

Cool, refreshing and packed full of antioxidants and nutrients, this smoothie is a great way to start your day.

The ingredients for this smoothie are:

- ½ avocado

- 2 dates

- juice of one lime

- 3 ice cubes

- one cup of coconut water

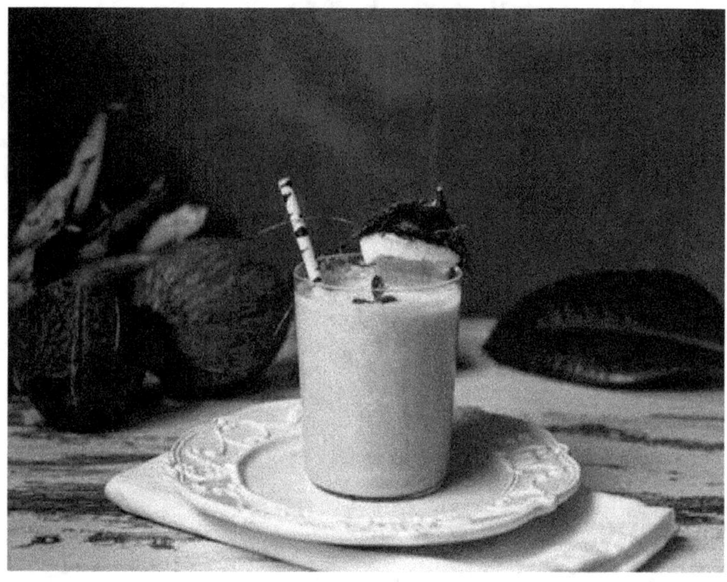

Add everything together into a high-speed blender and blend all together until a smooth consistency is reached. Serve cold.

This particular recipe is great for heart disease, diabetes, healthy skin, improving the immune system and nervous system, reducing constipation, and aiding weight loss!

Sprouted Buckwheat Crepes

To make this beautiful dish, very little ingredients are required, but the taste is fantastic, all while maintaining alkalinity.

Ingredients:
- one cup of buckwheat groat
- pure water
- ¼ cup of chia seeds
- 1 tsp vanilla extract

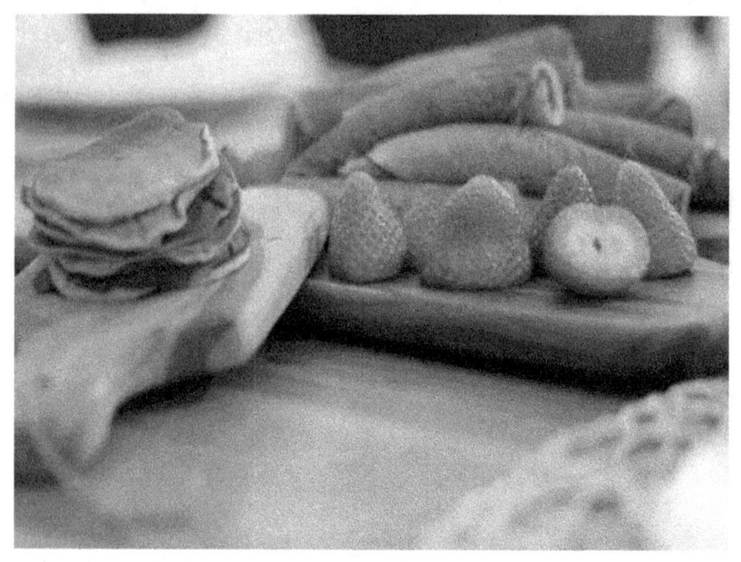

The directions to prepare this recipe include rinsing off your buckwheat really well and then soaking it in water until the morning. Place all the ingredients in the blender and process until it gets smooth. You will need to preheat your non-stick pan on a medium heat with coconut oil. Pour a thin layer of the mixture into the centre of the pan and swirl the pan in the right directions. When the crepe is browning, then you may cook it on the other side. Repeat it until the mixture is gone. Once all is done, then you may serve it properly to your audience and enjoy!

Healthy Baked Beans

Ingredients:

- two cups of cannellini beans (they must be rinsed and drained well)
- 1 can (6 oz.) tomato paste
- 1 white onion (diced)
- 1 clove garlic crushed
- 2 teaspoons smoked paprika
- 2 tbsp coconut oil
- 250g cherry tomatoes (halved)

To prepare, heat the pan on a low/medium heat with the coconut oil. Next, saute the onion and garlic until they are soft, and add the beans. Cook the cherry tomatoes and tomato paste for three minutes and add all

the seasoning, before serving it with spinach.
Enjoy!

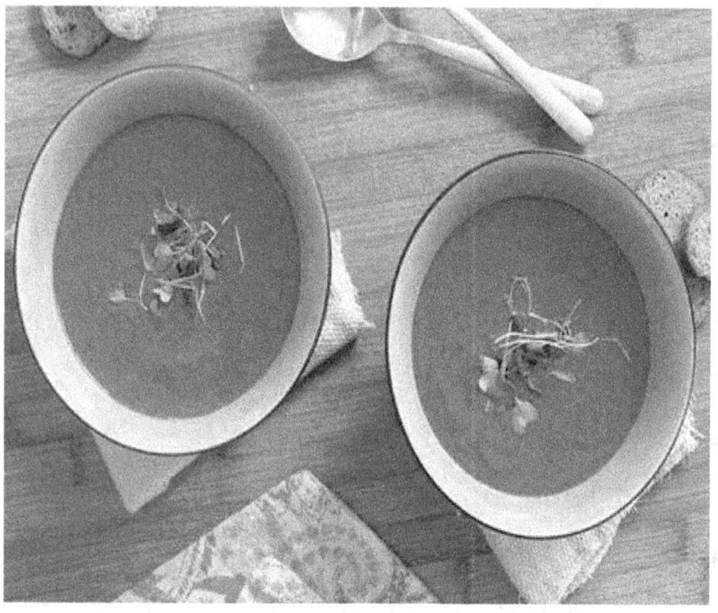

Grain-Free Granola

Ingredients:

- 70 g walnuts chopped

- 100g pumpkin seeds

- 100g sunflower seeds

- 60 g flaxseeds/linseeds

- 250g unsweetened coconut flakes

- 1 tsp ground ginger

- 50 g coconut oil

- 1 tsp ground cinnamon

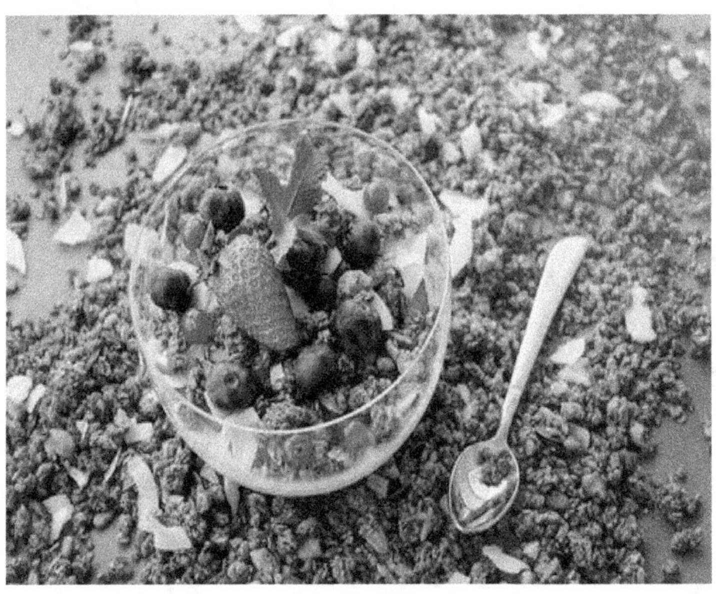

To create this fantastic recipe, add the nuts and seeds in a large roasting or baking dish with high sides. Mix thoroughly the nuts and seeds with cinnamon, ginger, coconut flakes and coconut oil with a large spoon or spatula.

Then bake at 180C/350F for 20 minutes. The mixture can burn very easily so you have to turn the mixture with the spatula every three minutes. The goal is to have the seeds and nuts toasted nicely. Next, allow to cool thoroughly and place in airtight containers. Enjoy!

Avocado Toasts

This recipe should be eaten regardless of time of day, because it's too good for time limitations! These toasts are the perfect dish for breakfast. Made with cherry tomatoes, this appetizer is sure to impress!

Ingredients:
- 1/2 baguette cut into thin slices
- 2 avocado
- 2 cups of cherry tomatoes

- 1 tbsp hemp oil

- Himalayan sea salt and pepper

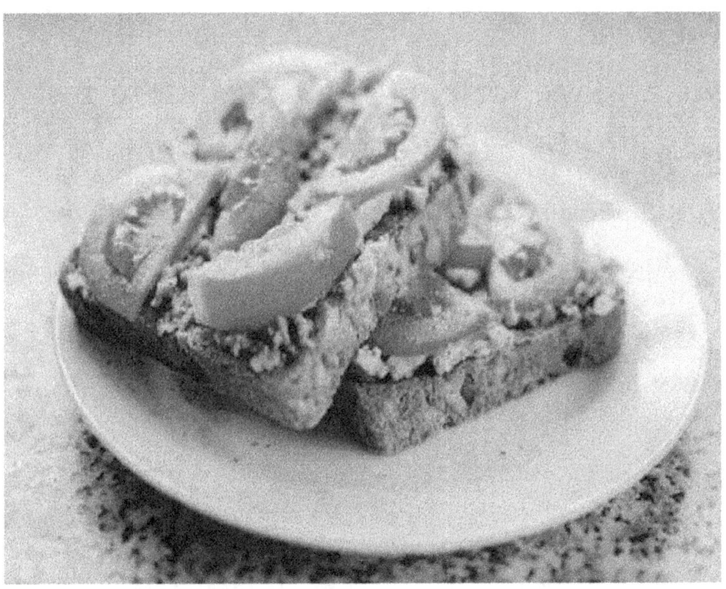

The directions include toasting your bread in the oven and then top with some cherry tomatoes, mashed avocado, Himalayan sea salt and pepper, and a minor drizzle of hemp oil for the tastiest and easiest breakfast!

These twelve different smoothies and easy recipes are good for you to eat in different situations, and great for you in all different ways, as they provide sheer alkalinity for your body. Not only that, but they're tasty, so you can get a great deal of enjoyment whilst eating them!

CHAPTER 12

30-Day Meal Plan

This chapter will discuss the transformation that takes place in the human body while eating alkaline foods. The previous chapters have clearly discussed the vitality of an alkaline diet, and have also given some extremely tasty recipes to you. You can have breakfast, lunch, dinner and also smoothie and other easy recipes while maintaining an alkaline PH within your body.

To help you become healthier, and achieve a better body shape, this chapter is recommending a 30-Day meal to you, and it is advised that each routine is followed carefully to achieve the comprehensive changes.

Day one

Breakfast – Strawberry Coco Chia Quinoa

The ingredients for this breakfast are one cup of cooked quinoa, 2 pitted dates, 5 tbsp. of chia seeds, 2 tbsp. of almond pieces, 1½ cup of almond, coconut or hemp milk, 2 tbsp. unsweetened shredded coconut flakes, 4 sliced strawberries and a ½ cup of quartered strawberries.

The results will be beneficial and have a high impact if you follow the recipe strictly. This recipe should be prepared the night before.

Cook quinoa and prepare other ingredients by mixing the strawberries, almond milk (or coconut/hemp milk) and two dates in a blender. Puree them until they are smoothed. Pour the mixture into a jar and add chia seeds to it. Then, mix until all the seeds are covered with the milk. Cover it with the lid, and then refrigerate overnight. In the morning, when you wake up, you must place the chia seeds in a bowl and add the quinoa in a uniformed manner. Serve with the shredded coconut and enjoy!

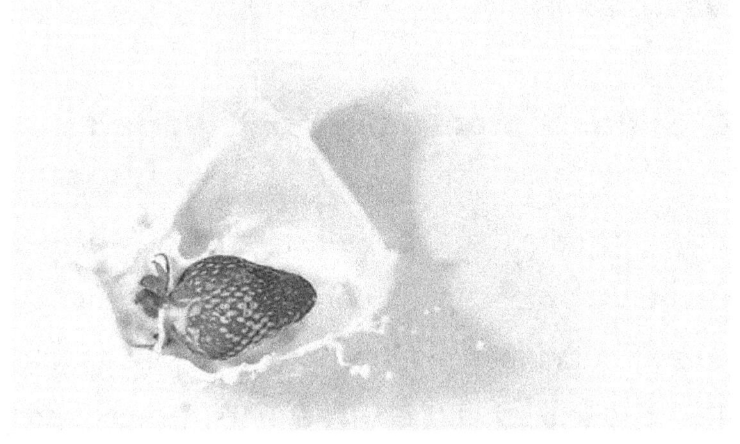

Lunch – Sweet and Savory Salad

The ingredients are one large head of butter lettuce, sliced cucumber, a cup of apple vinegar, one pomegranate, extra virgin oil, one avocado (cubed), one garlic clove and a quarter of a cup of shelled pistachios. The directions for this recipe are super simple! Hand tear the lettuce into a salad bowl, and then simply add the rest of the ingredients.

Day two

Breakfast – Non-Dairy Apple Parfait

The ingredients are half a cup of soaked cashews, one cup of chopped apple, half a cup of unsweetened almond or coconut milk, 1/3 cup rolled gluten-free oats (uncooked) and vanilla.

The directions are: add the cashews, almond milk (or coconut milk), and vanilla in a blender and blend until you reach a smooth consistency. The layering of the ingredients in a small cup is the next step. Heap a spoon of the cashew cream and dress the top with oats (the important last step to finish!).

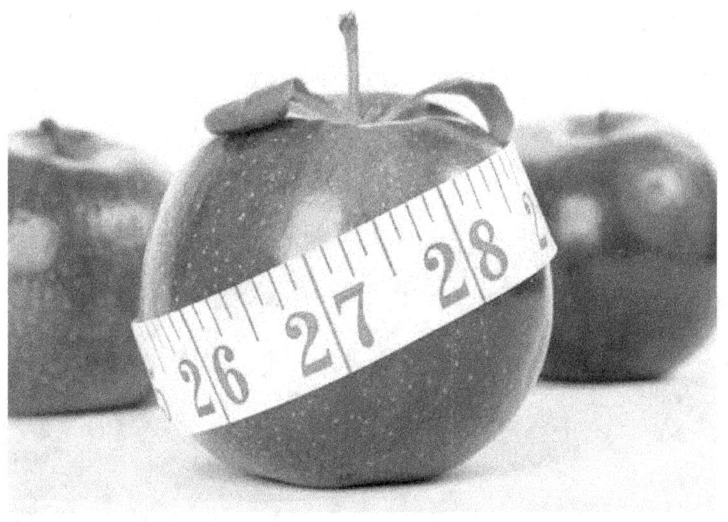

Lunch – Savoury Avocado Wrap

The ingredients for this recipe are 1 butter lettuce, 1 tablespoon of cilantro, ½ avocado, ¼ red onion, 1 tablespoon of chopped basil, a small handful of spinach and sea salt and pepper.

The directions for this recipe are: spread the avocado onto a leaf of the butter lettuce and sprinkle with salt, basil, cilantro, red onion and spinach. The final dressings really ensure the flavours of this dish come out!

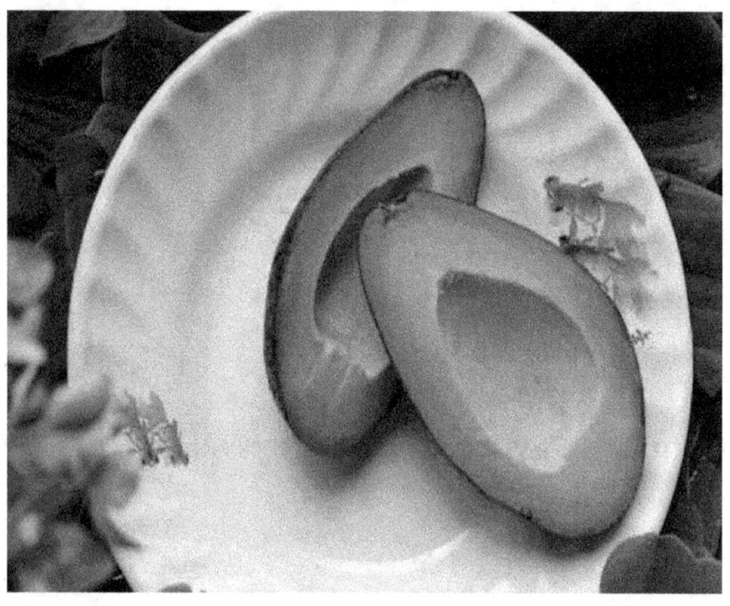

Day three

Breakfast – Almond Butter Crunch Berry Smoothie

The ingredients are two cups of fresh spinach, one banana (frozen), two cups of almond or coconut milk (unsweetened), four tbsp. of raw almond butter, one cup of any types of strawberries, grapes or mixed berries (frozen), and one tablespoon of chia seeds.

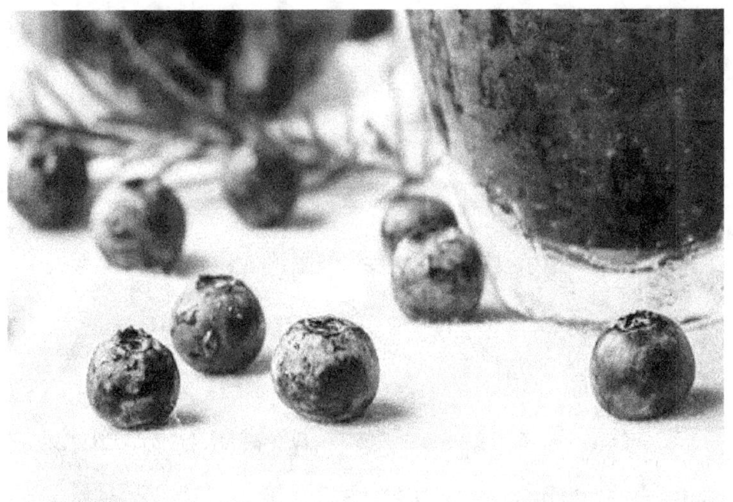

To prepare, blend the spinach and almond milk (or coconut milk) together first, before adding the remaining ingredients except for the chia seeds and blending again. Add the chia seeds once the mixture is smooth. Then, sit back and relax, and enjoy!

Lunch – Kale Pesto Zucchini Noodles

The ingredients for this recipe are one bunch kale (about 5 medium-large leaves, stems removed and roughly chopped), sea salt and pepper, two cups of fresh basil, one large green zucchini (spiralized or julienned), 3 – 4 tablespoon extra virgin olive oil (more as needed), half a cup of almonds, and, to garnish, sliced asparagus, spinach leaves, tomato, juice of 1 small lemon and a fresh sprinkle of salt.

To prepare this recipe, you should prepare the almonds the night before, by letting them soak. Then, when you are ready to eat, put all ingredients in the blender or food processor, and blend it until you get a nice creamy consistency. Lastly, add the zucchini noodles (you can use a spiralizer to get your curly noodle effect!).

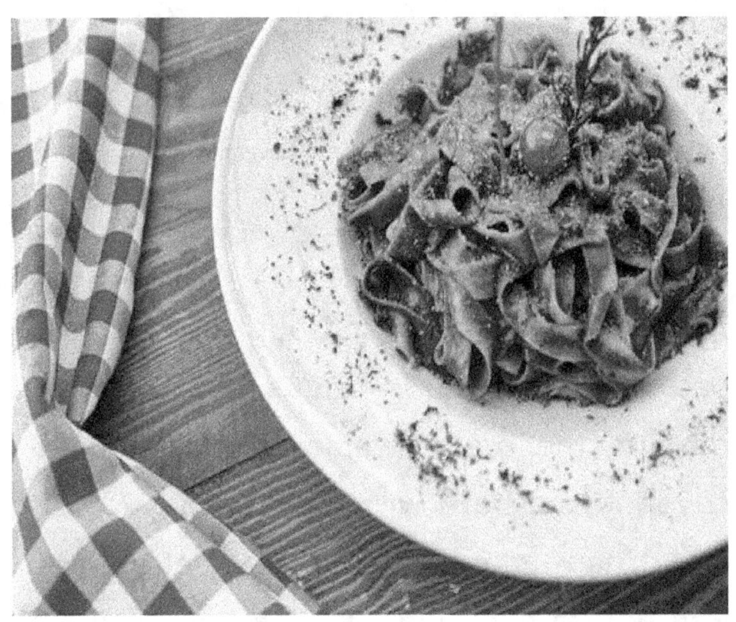

Day four

Breakfast – Apple and Almond Butter Oats

The ingredients to prepare this recipe include two cups of gluten-free oats, one cup of grated green apple, half a cup of coconut milk, ½ cup of yogurt, one teaspoon of cinnamon and 1/3 cup of almond butter.

The directions are: add the oats, coconut milk, yogurt and almond butter into a bowl and then mix well. After that, stir into the mixture the grated apple, and proceed by covering the bowl with a lid or plastic wrap and then place it in the refrigerator. Refrigerate overnight. If when you come to serve, the oats have become to thick in consistency for your liking, add some coconut milk. Finally, before serving, garnish with the cinnamon powder and enjoy!

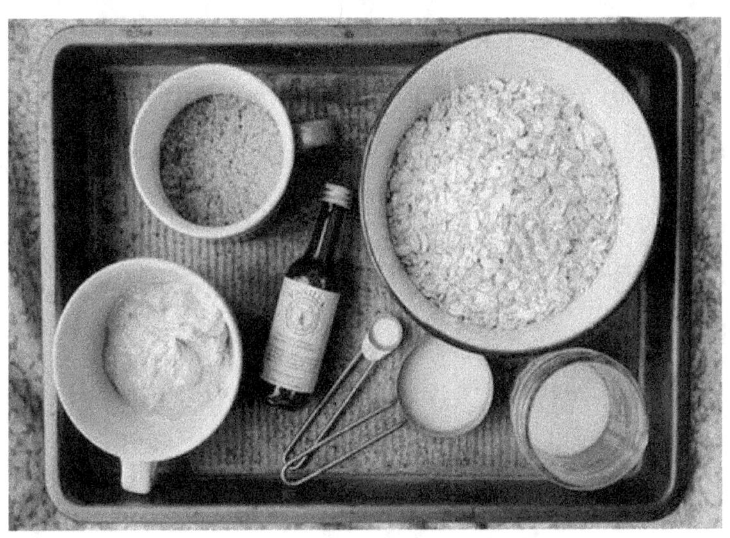

Lunch – Green Goddess Bowl with Avocado Cumin Dressing

The ingredients for this fantastic recipe are best sorted into three for your personal convenience:

For the Avocado Cumin Dressing, you will need one avocado, 1 tbsp. cumin powder, two limes, one cup of filtered water, a quarter of a tablespoon of sea salt, 1 tbsp. extra virgin olive oil, dash cayenne pepper, and a quarter of tsp. smoked paprika.

For the Tahini Lemon Dressing, you will need a quarter of a cup of tahini (sesame butter), half a cup of filtered water, half a lemon (freshly squeezed), one clove of minced garlic, ½ tsp. of sea salt, 1 tbsp. extra virgin olive oil, black pepper to taste.

For the salad, you will need three cups of kale (chopped), half a cup of kelp noodles, half a cup of broccoli florets (chopped), 1/3 cup of cherry tomatoes (halved), ½ zucchini (make noodles with spiralizer), and 2 tbsp. of hemp seeds.

To prepare this recipe, lightly steam kale and broccoli for four minutes, and then mix zucchini noodles and kelp noodles, before tossing with a generous serving of the smoked avocado and cumin dressing. Next, add the cherry tomatoes before tossing again. Then, plate the steamed kale and broccoli and drizzle with the Tahini Lemon Dressing, before topping the kale and broccoli with the dressed noodles and tomatoes. Finally, sprinkle the whole dish with the hemp seeds and enjoy!

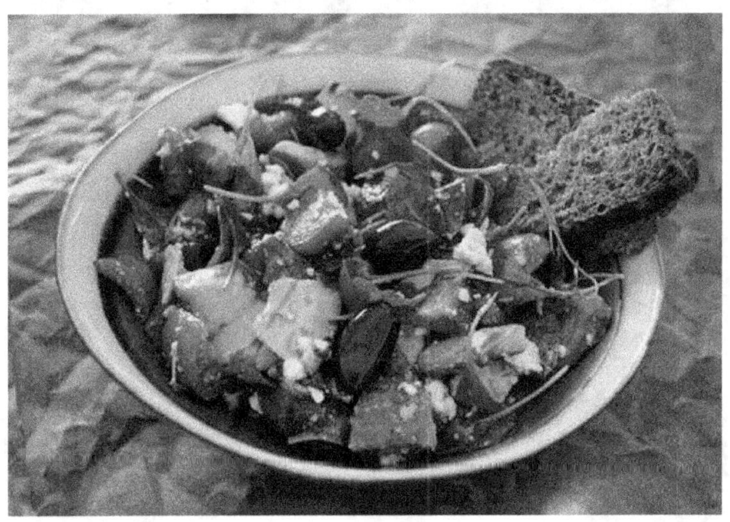

Day five

Breakfast – Berry Good Spinach Power Smoothie

The ingredients for this recipe are two cups of fresh spinach, two tbsp. of coconut oil, two cups of unsweetened almond milk, ½ tsp. of cinnamon, one cup of mixed berries (frozen), 1 tbsp. of raw almond butter and one frozen banana.

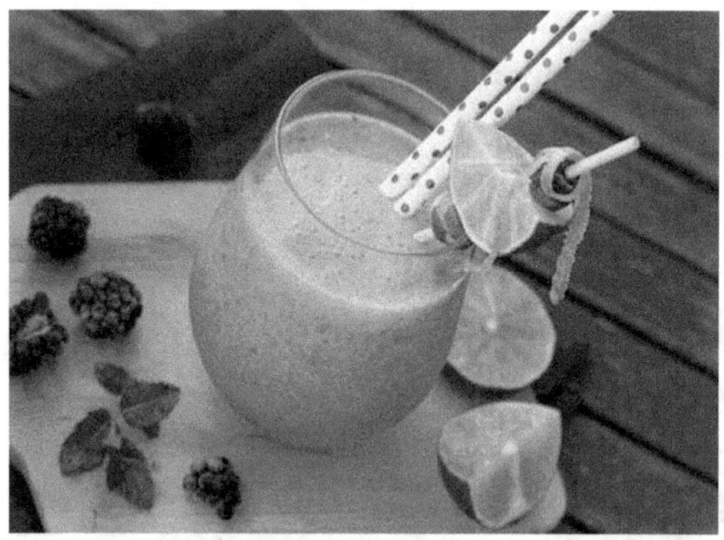

The directions for preparing this recipe is, firstly, blend the spinach and almond milk. Then, you can add the remaining ingredients to the mixture, and blend again until reaching your desired consistency.

Lunch – Quinoa Burrito Bowls

The ingredients for this recipe are a cup of quinoa, one clove garlic minced, one tbsp of extra virgin olive oil, two hundred and fifty grams of black beans (drained & rinsed), one teaspoon of ground cumin, one teaspoon of dried oregano, two red onions (sliced), two avocados (sliced), 1/2 teaspoon of sea salt, 1/2 cup of chopped fresh cilantro and two limes (freshly juiced).

The directions for preparing this recipe are to first cook the quinoa (pour the quinoa into a saucepan along with 2 cups of water and then bring the quinoa to a boil) and beans (in a small saucepan, cook the black beans with the extra virgin olive oil, onions and minced garlic, over medium heat, then combine with the cumin and oregano). When the quinoa is finished cooking, add cilantro and lime juice. Then, divide the mixture into various serving bowls, before finally topping with the beans and avocado sliced.

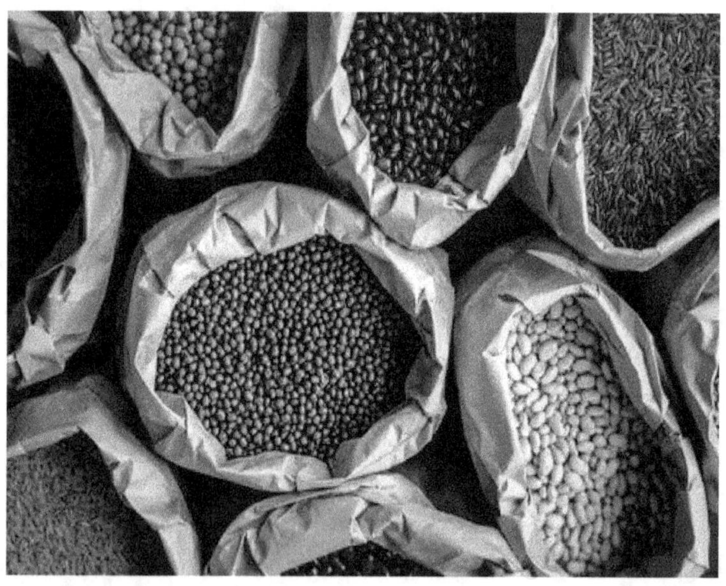

Day six

Breakfast – Quinoa Morning Porridge

The ingredients for this tasty recipe are half a cup of rinsed quinoa, chia seeds, a can of coconut milk, hemp seeds, and cinnamon. The directions are super simple! Add all of the ingredients, except the hemp seeds, and simmer them for 10-15 minutes until all of the liquid is absorbed. Then, to serve, top with the hemp seeds.

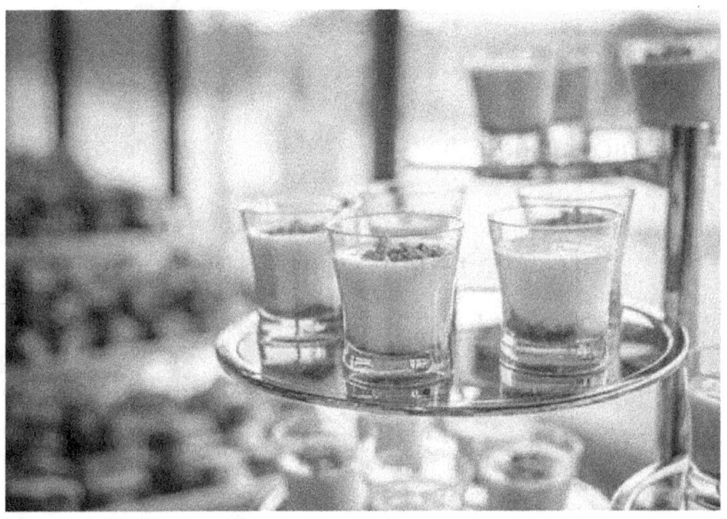

Lunch – Thai Quinoa Salad

The ingredients will be split into two, both the dressing and the salad, for your convenience. The ingredients for the dressing are chopped seeds, a cup of tahini (it's a paste made from toasted and ground sesame seeds), a lemon (freshly juiced), one pitted date, one teaspoon of apple cider vinegar, salt, one tamari (it is a Japanese sauce made of fermented soybeans), and sesame oil.

The ingredients for the salad are one cup of quinoa (steamed), one tomato (sliced), one large handful of arugula, and a quarter of a red onion (sliced).

To prepare this recipe, blend the ingredients together to make the dressing.

Then, steam one cup of quinoa in a steamer or rice cooker, and then set aside. After, prepare the other ingredients for the salad, and then add together a combination of all the quinoa, arugula, sliced tomatoes, and sliced red onion. Afterwards, serve on a plate or in a salad bowl and garnish with the Thai Dressing beforehand mixing with a spoon and enjoy!

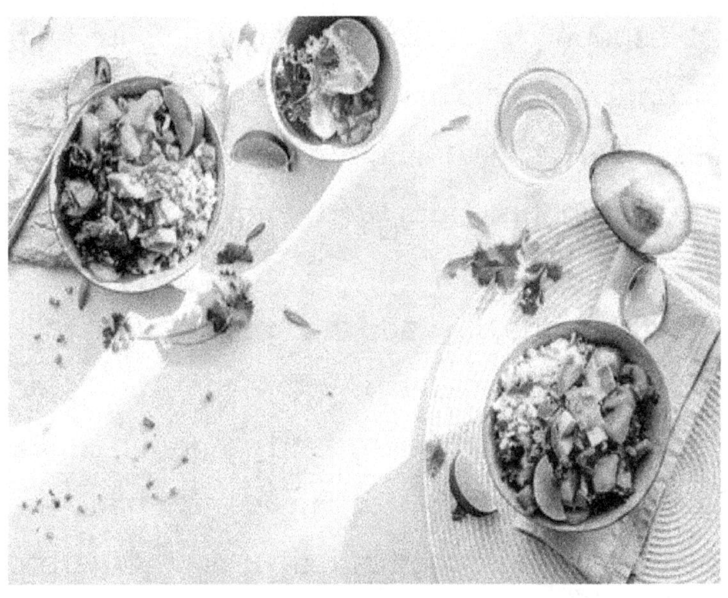

Day seven

Breakfast – Alkaline Warrior Chia Breakfast

The ingredients for this breakfast are one cup of unsweetened almond or coconut milk, one tablespoon of unsweetened shredded coconut flakes, three tablespoons of chia seeds, ½ tsp. vanilla, ½ tsp. cinnamon, ½ cup of chopped nuts, and one tbsp. of hemp seeds.

The directions are: add a combination of milk and chia seeds together into a jar. Then, add the vanilla, cinnamon, and chopped nuts. Next, cover the jar with the lid and shake the mixture until it's combined; then refrigerate overnight. In the morning, when you are ready to serve, shake or stir, and divide into one or two bowls. Top with fresh fruit, coconut shreds, and if you choose, with more chopped nuts.

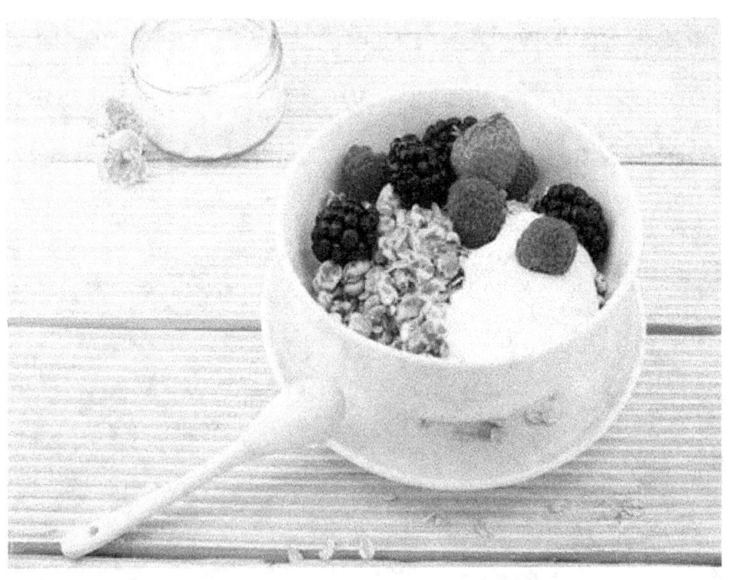

Lunch - Asian Sesame Dressing and Noodles

The ingredients for this recipe are one tablespoon of tahini (sesame butter), one tsp. of tamari (gluten-free), one tsp. of liquid coconut nectar, a lemon (freshly squeezed), one scallion (chopped), one tablespoon of sesame seeds, a sliced red bell pepper and a sliced yellow bell pepper. For the noodles, you can choose between either zucchini noodles or kelp noodles.

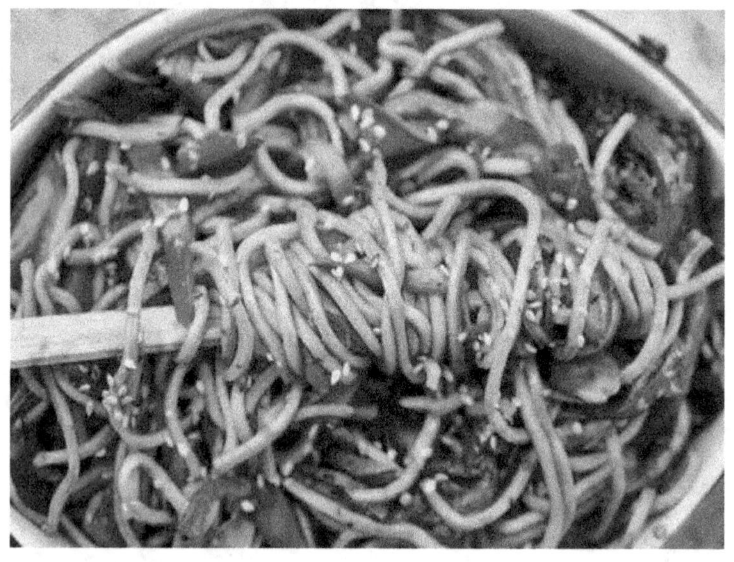

The directions for preparing this lunch are: in a bowl, combine all the dressing ingredients and thoroughly mix with a spoon. To make zucchini noodles, use a spiralizer or, if you are using kelp noodles, place them in warm water for five minutes to rinse off the liquid then are packaged in, and allow them to separate and soften. Add the dressing to the noodles and mix thoroughly. Then, add sesame seeds, serve and enjoy!

Day Eight

Breakfast – French Toast

The ingredients for this recipe are just simply bread and egg!

This breakfast is widely shared and eaten throughout the world. French toast has all the necessary ingredients that boost energy within your body, and the ingredients are especially alkaline in their nature, thus promoting better health. The ingredients for this simple and tasty recipe are 1 egg, ¼ cup of milk, 4 slices bread, 1 teaspoon of vanilla extract and 1/2 teaspoon of ground cinnamon. To prepare this tasty breakfast you have to beat egg, vanilla and cinnamon in a dish and then stir in milk. The next step is to dip bread in the mixture and then cook bread slices on the skillet on medium heat until browned on both sides. You can serve with maple syrup if desired!

Lunch – Summer Salad with Citrus Dressing

Lunch will be the summer salad with citrus dressing. Salads make a fantastic lunch and extremely useful in maintaining an alkaline diet to improve health. To reap the best possible benefits, try to mix tomatoes, carrots, green leaf, cabbage and lemons (juice) into the salad.

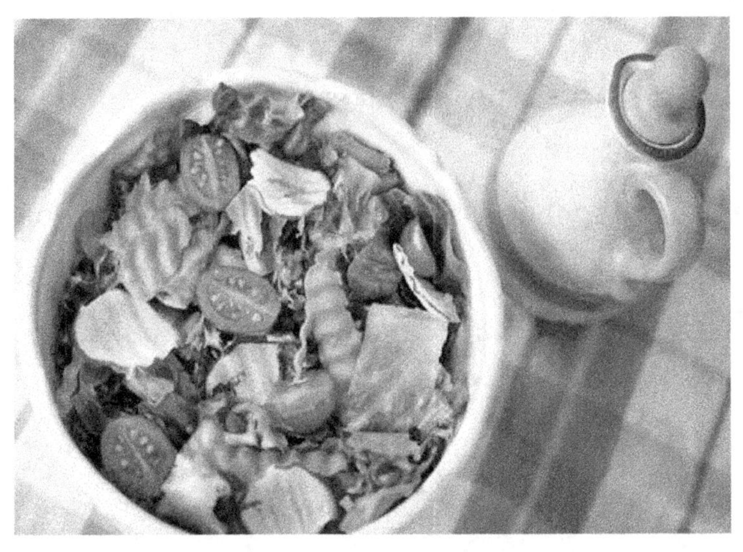

If you prefer a more salty taste, you can sprinkle some Himalayan sea salt on the salad for your enjoyment! This meal is beneficial in aiding in better health, and can be used in many situations where you want a quick lunch, but want the fantastic results that an alkaline diet can give you!

Day Nine

Breakfast- Apple Pancakes

Apple pancakes are a great treasure for you if you strive for an alkaline diet, and with a cup of tea, apple pancakes are actually one of the healthiest alkaline meals of all.

A beautiful mix of apples in the sweet aroma of cake batter, these pancakes are very easy to make and they can be given in a range of different prices to customers.

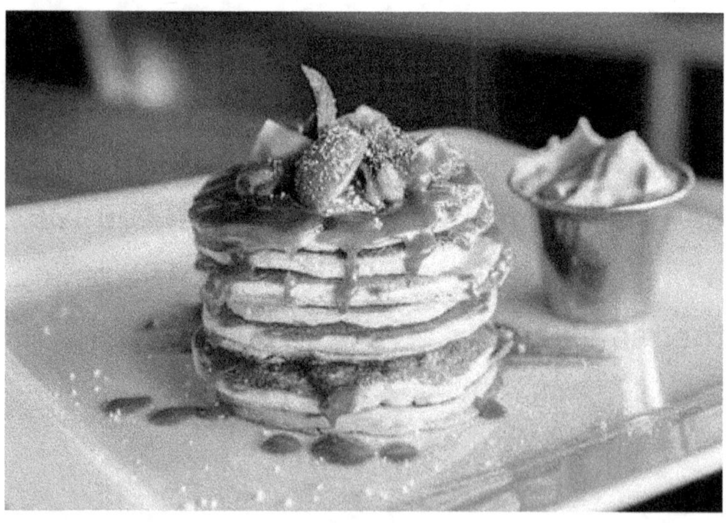

To make them, you will need: 1½ cups of flour, 2 tablespoons of sugar, ¼ teaspoon of grounded cinnamon, 2 eggs (whisked), 2 teaspoons of baking powder, 1 teaspoon of baking soda, ½ teaspoon of salt, 1¼ cup of milk, two red apples (shredded), ¼ cup of applesauce, cooking oil (if necessary), blueberries and low-fat frozen yogurt. With these simple ingredients, apple pancakes can be easily made and there is a lot of delicious taste attached to them.

The directions for preparing this breakfast are: in a large bowl, sift together flour, sugar, baking powder, baking soda and salt. Whisk in milk, eggs, applesauce, and cinnamon just until combined; stir in shredded apples. Preheat a flat griddle over medium-high heat. Pour ¼ cup of pancake batter onto the griddle. Let pancakes cook until bubbles form before flipping.

Cook the other side until golden brown. Serve hot with syrup and, if you want, you can add blueberries (or other fruits) and low-fat frozen yogurt.

Lunch - Cheesy Kale Chips and Sliced Fruit

This recipe contains all the necessary amount of minerals, amino acids, proteins, and enzymes the human body needs! It's also straightforward to make and provide a lot of energy! This recipe also contains a sliced portion of fruit for you! Fruit, coupled with these chips, can be very prolific for your health. Like this, you could achieve all the accumulation of satisfaction, in both body and mind that you could get!

The ingredients for this tasty recipe are: 8 cups of kale and 2 cups of raw vegan cheese

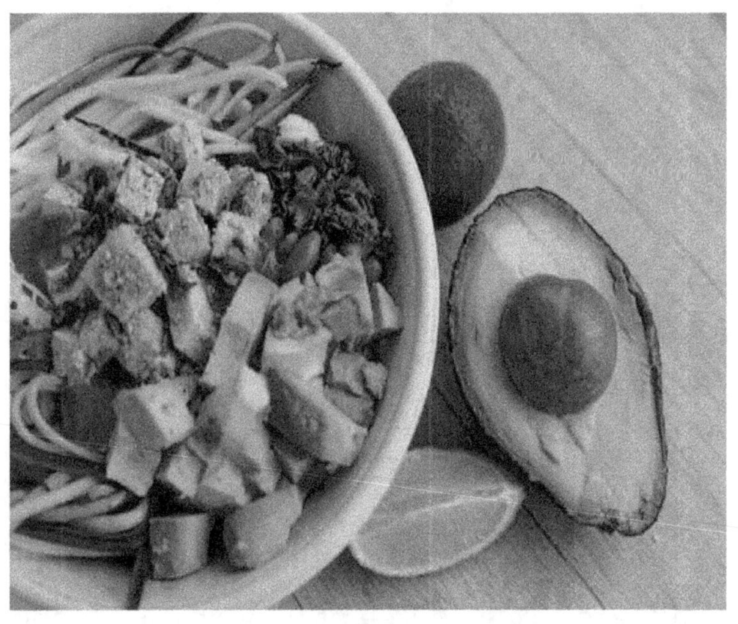

Its ingredients are a handful of corn tortilla chips (crumbled), half a spoon of firm tofu, one ripe avocado (peeled, pitted and sliced), one cup of halved cherry tomatoes (optional), a handful of almonds (or walnuts, or any other nuts), one spoon of chili sauce, a generous handful of chopped fresh cilantro, half a red onion, sea salt, pepper and half a lemon (fresh lemon juice).

It is incredibly simple to make, and perfect for anyone who wants a fast but extremely healthy diet!

Lunch - Green Beans with Toasted Almonds

An almond contains infinite pieces of energy for your body! Green beans, on the other hand, are a rich source of vitamins A, C, and K, and of folic acid and fiber.

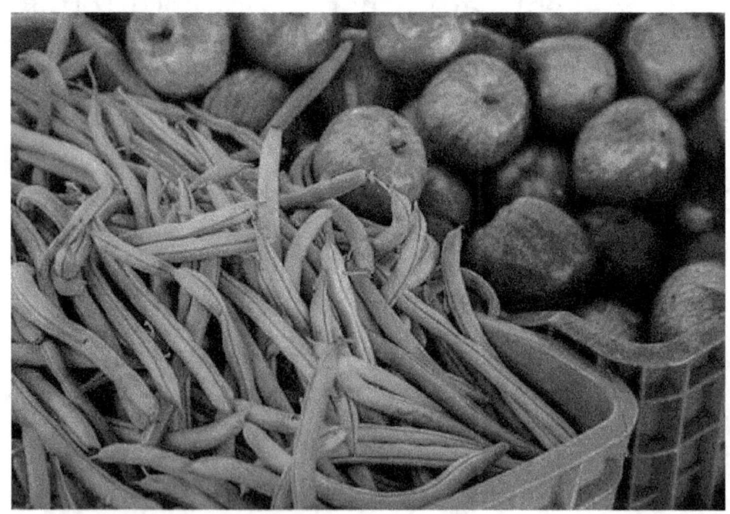

The ingredients to prepare this delicious recipe are: 1 lb. of green beans (skinny French String beans), 2 tbsp. of coconut oil, 2 cloves garlic (minced), 1/2 cup of sliced almonds, 1 tablespoon of fresh lemon juice, sea salt to taste (Celtic Grey, Himalayan, or Redmond Real Salt). The directions are: in a large pot of boiling water blanch green beans for 2-3 minutes. Then, remove from heat, drain well and dry with paper towels. Done this, in a large skillet over medium-low heat add the coconut oil and sliced almonds and cook for 2-3 minutes. Then add green beans and garlic and cook for 5-6 minutes tossing frequently. At the end add lemon juice and serve. Now you're ready to enjoy this fantastic and healthy recipe!

Day eleven

Breakfast – Mixed Sprouts Salad

If you want to start your day with a tasteful alkaline diet then mixed sprouts is the best salad for you! It has a large number of proteins, vitamins, minerals and energy, which is extremely beneficial for you!

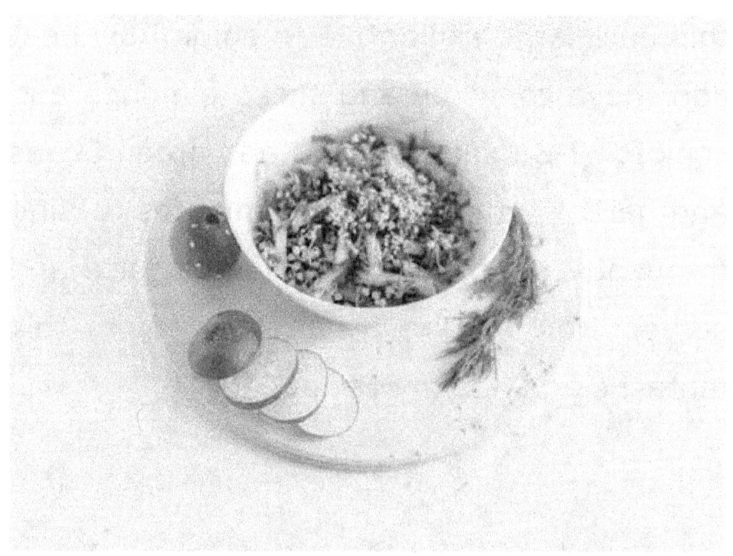

Its ingredients include fifty grams of sprouts, one cup of cucumber (peeled and cubed), one cup of chopped spring onions, a handful of parsley, fresh juice of a lemon, Celtic sea salt, and black pepper. The making of it is also very basic (combine all ingredients in a salad bowl), and it helps to give you the best amount of energy you can possibly achieve.

Lunch – Red cabbage, Beetroot & Apple Salad

This salad is very alkaline in its nature and can be helpful throughout the entire year! The ingredients to prepare this tasty and healthy recipe are: one apple (cored and finely sliced), 500g of red cabbage (thinly sliced), 100g of raw beetroot (peeled and finely grated), 1 tbsp of cider vinegar, 2 tbsp extra-virgin olive oil, 30g of pomegranate seeds, fresh juice of a lemon, sea salt to taste and small bunch parsley (chopped). The directions are very easy: combine all the ingredients in a large salad bowl and then serve!

The beetroot can condense the fat intake into proper chemicals that can then be helpful for your body. You can then stay alert in your busy routine throughout the year, and you can relish in your newly found elevated energy levels! You will, for example, be able to give proper satisfaction to your clients any way in your daily duty. You can strive for excellence and betterment in all ways possible. You will feel great and have an enormous amount of excellency in your lifestyle.

Day twelve

Breakfast – Kale Chickpea Mash

This dish, with its name, sounds delicious, and, better yet, it provides all the necessary benefits for you!

The ingredients to make it are two tablespoons of garlic (minced), one shallot (minced), one bunch of kale, three hundred grams of fresh chickpeas, two tablespoons of coconut oil (or extra virgin olive oil) and Himalayan sea salt for more relish. The making of this recipe is also effortless. You just need to fry the shallot and minced garlic in coconut oil. Then, wait until it turns golden brown, and then you can add the kale (washed and drained). Now add the chickpeas and start to cook them, too (for about five minutes). In the end, add the remaining ingredients, stir and then mash the chickpeas with a fork. Your dish is finally ready to be served!

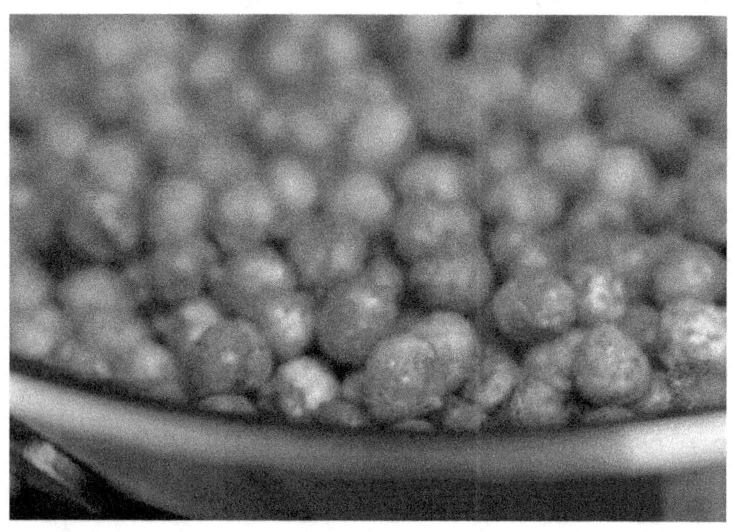

Lunch – Zucchini Sushi

The zucchini sushi will be just the lunch for you if you are a sushi lover and want to maintain an alkaline state to your body!
You can get all the enjoyment while making it, and your body will be able to perform well after eating it. The ingredients for this

fabulous alkaline recipe are four zucchini (sliced), a quarter cup of parsley (minced), two artichoke hearts (cut in small pieces), two cloves of garlic (minced), one lemon (freshly juiced) and one can of white beans. You can slice the juicy zucchini in any way you choose, before mixing all the ingredients in a medium bowl for all possible tastes and flavours and maximum enjoyment!

Day thirteen

Breakfast – Quinoa and Apple Breakfast

This breakfast food you will really enjoy, as it has only the finest ingredients! The ingredients are a half cup of quinoa, one large apple (cut in pieces), and two teaspoons of cinnamon. These ingredients will produce the most excellent alkaline breakfast for you that will have all the healthy proteins, enzymes and vitamins you need! To create it, you have to cook the quinoa first (you have to add some water, and it is advised to boil the water for fifteen minutes). Next, add the apple and cook for thirty seconds, before sprinkling some cinnamon. You can add some optional raisins for an elegant taste.

Lunch - Courgette and Quinoa Salad

The ingredients of this salad are very healthy for your body. They are: 300g of courgettes (washed and sliced), ½ cup of quinoa, 1 tsp of cumin, 400g of tin chickpeas (which are rinsed well and drained), 1 garlic clove (which is crushed with sea salt), 2 tablespoons of extra virgin olive oil, 2 tablespoons of lemon juice, 2 spring onions (chopped), and a small handful of flat-leaf parsley leaves (chopped). The directions to create this tasty recipe are really simple. Add the quinoa to a pot, then add a cup of water, and bring to the boil over medium heat before simmering it for ten minutes or until all the water is absorbed. Replace the lid and prepare all the other ingredients. After doing it, heat the extra virgin olive oil in a large pan. Addition of the courgettes is the next step. While cooking, stir until bright green and tender. Spoon into a bowl, season and then set aside. Replace the pan over medium heat; add the cumin and cook, stirring until fragrant. In the last step, add the chickpeas, quinoa, garlic, lemon juice, spring onions, and parsley and toss well. Now, you're ready to serve!

Day fourteen

Breakfast – Cold Oats

This cold dish is a fantastic breakfast alkaline food for you that can give to your metabolism a tremendous boost! The ingredients of this meal contain half a cup of oats, half a cup of milk (you can choose your favorite milk!), half a cup of yoghurt, a pinch of salt, half a teaspoon of cinnamon, one banana (sliced), half a cup of berries and one tbsp of chia seeds (or other seeds, as you prefer!). You can replace the banana and the berries with other fruit of your choice (like, for example, strawberries). Instead, if you want a vegan recipe, you can choose nondairy yogurt and milk (options include almond, cashew, soy, rice, oat, or coconut).

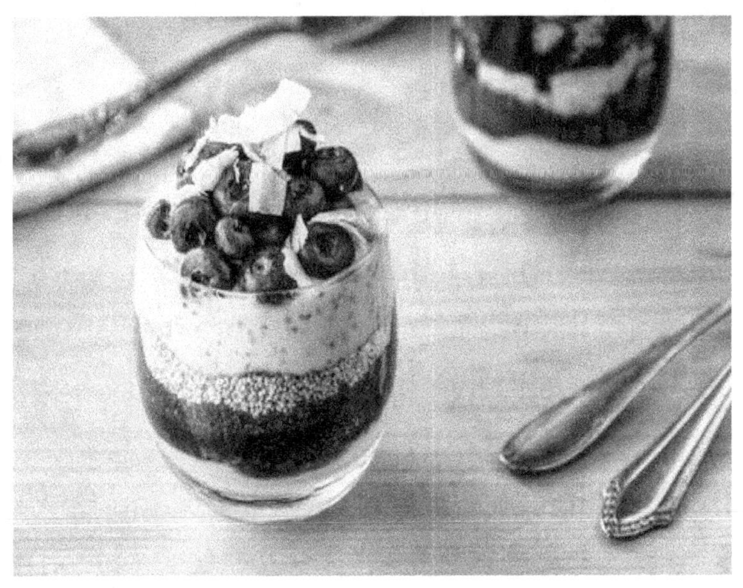

The steps to preparing it are also straightforward to understand. Combine all ingredients in a jar, then shake well and refrigerate overnight. The next morning, simply stir, so it's absolutely delicious!

Lunch – Cauliflower Gnocchi

This dish is vegan and excellent in its creation. The ingredients include one head of cauliflower (steamed or boiled), one garlic clove (chopped), one cup of flour, one tablespoon of olive or coconut oil to fry.

Instead, for the ragout, you need one tin of whole tomatoes, four courgettes (sliced), half an onion (finely sliced), one tablespoon of olive or coconut oil, one garlic clove (chopped), five large black mushrooms (sliced), three hundred milliliters of vegetable stock and one tsp of sugar. In the end, salt to taste and fresh basil to serve.

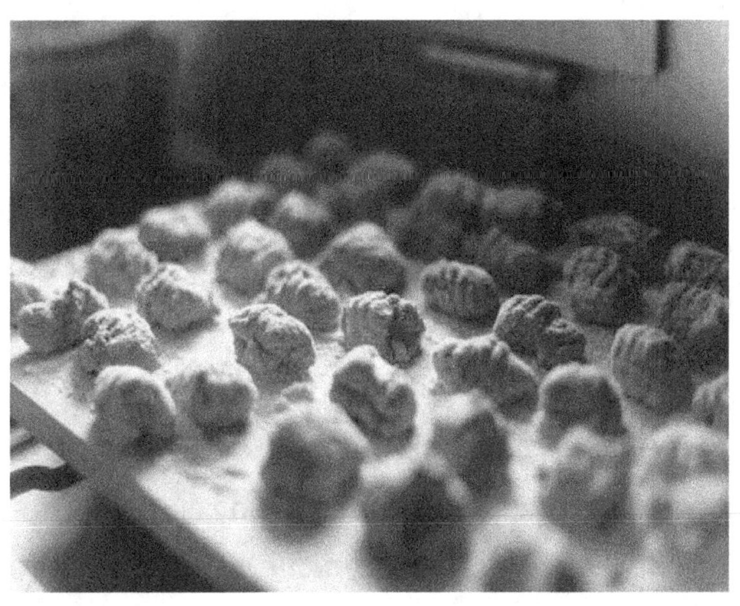

The directions to prepare this delicious recipe are: place the cauliflower and garlic in a blender (or food processor) and blend until smooth. Then, add a little water (if needed), salt and flour (1/4 cup at a time) and continue to process until a soft dough is formed. Turn out on a floured surface and knead briefly until dough is soft. Cut dough into four pieces, take one and roll out into a rope approximately 3 cm, then cut into 3cm pieces (after doing it, repeat with remaining dough). Now you're ready for cooking: place the olive oil (or coconut oil) in a non-stick pan and fry the gnocchi until lightly browned on both sides. Instead, for the ragout, place the olive oil (or coconut oil) in a non-stick pot over medium-high heat. Add the onion, garlic, mushrooms and courgettes and fry until starting to colour and soften. Add the tomatoes, vegetable stock and sugar, reduce to medium heat and allow to gently simmer for 20 minutes - until the vegetables are tender. Serve the ragout with the warm cauliflower gnocchi on top and then scattered with basil leaves.

Like this, a protein-enriched alkaline diet is at your service, and will yield you fantastic results for your health!

Day fifteen

Breakfast – Scrambled Tofu

Let's assume for one minute that you are a corporate business owner and you have to leave early for your job. For an extremely good lifestyle and great attention, the best possible breakfast that you can have is scrambled tofu! Its ingredients have a fantastic taste, and therefore, you can relish in all the energizing benefits but also still enjoy its consumption!

The ingredients are one onion (finely diced), one garlic clove (minced), three tomatoes (sliced), 1/2 package of firm tofu (very well-drained, but not pressed!), half a teaspoon of ground cumin, half a teaspoon of paprika, half a teaspoon of turmeric, one teaspoon of nutritional yeast, 2/3 cup of filtered water,

150g of baby spinach and a pinch of sea salt (or black salt, also known as "Kala Namak").

The steps to preparing this meal are: in a bowl combine turmeric, cumin, paprika, water, nutritional yeast and salt. Then add onion and garlic into a frying pan, and saute until fragrant (about 1-2 minutes). After doing this, crumble tofu into the pan (use your hands to break up the block of tofu) and pour the seasoning over tofu (it's necessary to mix well). Cook for 3 minutes or until tofu is hot throughout. Once cooked, add the tomatoes and the baby spinach, and this late addition will make the taste absolutely divine!

Lunch – Kale and Cucumber Kimchi

Kimchi is a popular Korean side dish, packed with beneficial nutrients. In short words, kimchi is a fermented vegetable dish. In this way, it is very beneficial and healthy for you. It gives you a great amount of protein, amino acids and triggers pro-active digestion in your body, because the vegetables are fermented, so they have excellent probiotic qualities. This dish can help you with conditions like inflammation and digestive issues.

The ingredients of this particular recipe are 250g of white cabbage (sliced), 250g of kale (chopped), 250g of cucumber (diced), sea salt, 2 tbsp. of dried chili flakes, 1 tbsp. of smoked paprika, 3 garlic cloves (minced), 1 tbsp. of fresh ginger (finely grated) and 500ml of mineral water.

The directions to prepare this healthy recipe are: combine the cabbage, kale, cucumber and salt together, then squeeze the vegetables, with your hands, for five minutes. With this method, natural water can easily come out of the vegetables and will provide a great amount of taste. After doing this, stir in the rest of the ingredients and transfer it to a sterilized jar with a lid.

Tips: leave it on the kitchen counter, away from direct sunlight, and fermentation of the mixture will take place (the recommended time is three weeks before tasting). Transfer it to the fridge once you are ready with the taste.

Day sixteen

Breakfast – Theplas

In the southern states of the Punjab region, Pakistan, and India, this recipe (theplas) is a Gujarati meal that is very alkaline in its creation. The ingredients of this delicious recipe are: 1 teaspoon of coriander powder, 1 tablespoon of curd (yogurt), 1 teaspoon of red chilli powder, 1/2 teaspoon of turmeric powder, 1/2 cup of finely chopped spinach leaves (optional), 1/4 teaspoon of carom seeds (or sesame seeds), 1 cup + 1/2 cup of wheat flour, 2 teaspoons of oil (+ for shallow frying), salt and water.

These ingredients will create a perfect breakfast addition to your alkaline diet plan; however, some care is needed while preparing it!

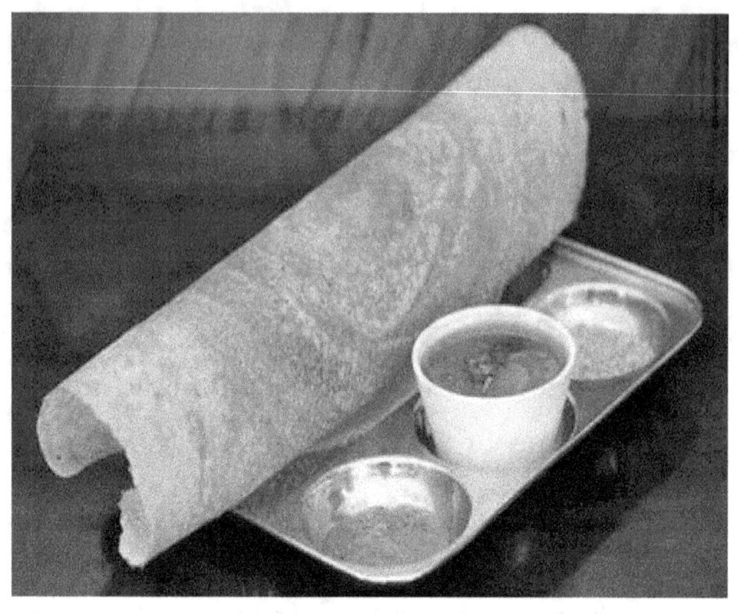

The steps to prepare this dish are: first combine in a bowl one cup of wheat flour, spinach leaves, curd, red chilli powder, coriander powder, turmeric powder, 1 teaspoon of oil and salt. Next, add water as needed in small incremental quantities and knead a smooth and soft dough. After doing this, cover the dough with a plate and leave aside for 15-20 minutes. Then, divide it into seven equal parts. Now, take 1/2 cup of dry wheat flour in a plate for dusting. Take one dough ball, press it against the rolling board to flatten it and transform into a circle having approx. 6-7 inch diameter. Heat the griddle over medium flame and when it's hot, place raw thepla on it. When tiny bubbles appear on the top surface, flip it over and cook for 30 seconds. Flip it again, and cook the other side as well. Repeat the flip-cook process until light golden brown spots appear on both sides. Transfer it to a plate, then follow the same process for remaining dough balls. Gujarati theplas are now ready. Enjoy!

Lunch – Cauliflower Tabbouleh Salad

This dish is very alkaline and thus is extremely beneficial for your health.

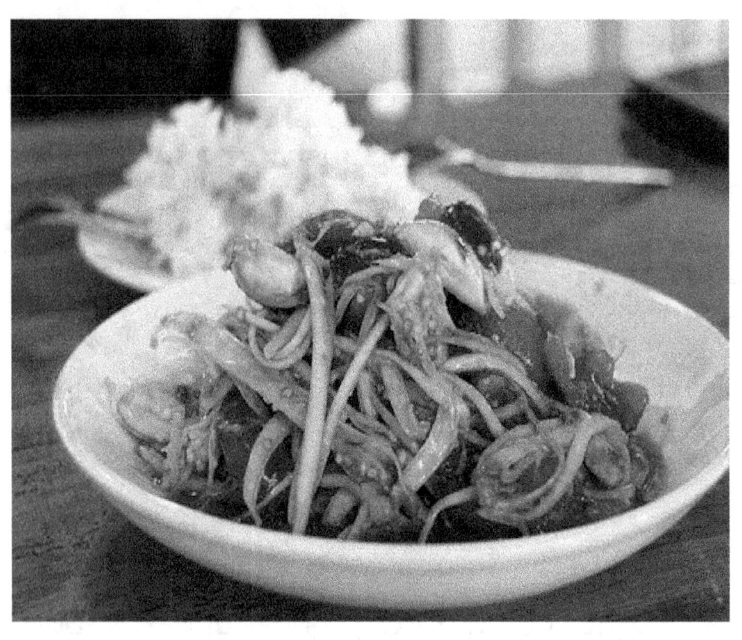

The ingredients to prepare this tasty recipe are: one raw head of cauliflower (coarsely chopped), two onions (chopped), 2 cups (packed) of flat-leaf parsley leaves with tender stems (minced), 1 cup (packed) of mint leaves (minced), ½ cucumber (finely diced), 150g of cherry tomatoes (quartered), 1 garlic clove (coarsely chopped), 1/4 teaspoon of crushed red pepper flakes, 3 tablespoons of extra-virgin olive oil, and sea salt to taste. In the end, the juice of one small lemon will add that little bit more flavour!

The method is very crucial, as, in a tabbouleh salad, the cauliflower must be dried, washed and cut correctly. Cut the cauliflower into chunks and add it into a food processor. Any process of cutting it down is ok, but it needs to be extremely fine in its consistency. Now, for cooking the cauliflower, heat the pan over medium heat. Add a bit of extra virgin olive oil, and cook the cauliflower until brown (continue heating and stirring until cauliflower starts to release some of its moisture and is crisp-tender). When cauliflower is cool, place in a large salad bowl with cucumber, tomatoes, onions, garlic, red pepper flakes, extra virgin olive oil, sea salt, mint and parsley. Then, add the lemon juice for a fresh and authentic taste!

Day seventeen

Breakfast – Maple Millet Porridge

A diet filled with proteins and amino acids awaits you!

The ingredients for this delicious breakfast are one cup of millet, two cups of filtered water, one cup of unsweetened coconut milk, a pinch of salt, 1/4 tsp of cinnamon and maple syrup to taste. All these ingredients can be very prolific for the human body!

To prepare this fantastic alkaline breakfast, first, put the millet in a food processor and blend. Then add the processed millet in a saucepan with the milk, maple syrup, water, and cinnamon. Bring to the boil then turn the heat down to simmer and cook for around 15 minutes until it is very creamy. Serve in a bowl when it is ready and, if you want, top with fresh raspberries (100g) and pumpkin seeds (1 teaspoon).

It is highly encouraged to enjoy this breakfast often and incorporate it into your lifestyle, as not only is it delicious, but it is also incredibly easy to cook. You can have all the joy of eating great food, but also reap the benefits of maintaining an alkaline body state at the same time.

Lunch - Grilled Courgette Salad

The best alkaline dish that you can taste for maintaining a healthy body is a grilled courgette salad! There are spicy ingredients too that can slightly boost metabolism, increasing the number of calories you burn throughout the day.

The ingredients to prepare this easy recipe are: six courgettes, one red chilli, one handful of fresh mint leaves, extra virgin olive oil, freshly ground black pepper and sea salt.

To prepare this fantastic meal, slice the courgettes lengthwise (as thin as you can) and then grill on a griddle pan (or on the barbecue), until lightly charred on each side. Scatter the slices over a large plate and then sprinkle them with a little sea salt and freshly ground black pepper. Now, wash the mint leaves and red chilli and chop finely, then sprinkle the chilli and mint evenly from a height over the courgettes. To finish, drizzle with good extra virgin olive oil. All these ingredients will create an intense flavour experience for you to enjoy!

Day eighteen

Breakfast – Beetroot Latte

Today's breakfast will be beetroot latte. Beetroot latte can be very helpful for your body as it provides an enormous amount of energy! If you also add one cup of almond milk in the latte, it will be beneficial for you. The beetroot latte is also very colourful, and it is lovely and creamy. It combines all the best ingredients and even helps regulate blood pressure; this recipe is very easy to prepare!

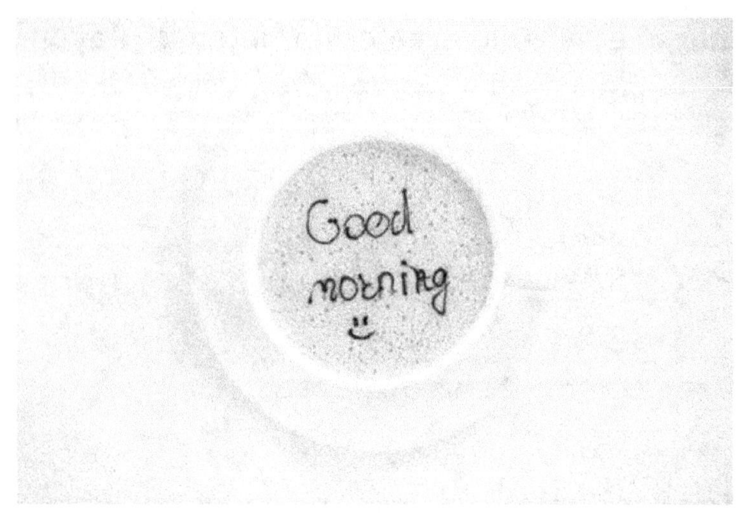

The ingredients to prepare beetroot latte are: one shot of fresh beetroot juice (or two teaspoons of beet powder), one teaspoon of honey (it's important to use a good quality of honey, better if it's organic!), one cup of unsweetened almond milk, and a sprinkle of cinnamon (this ingredient is optional). Now warm the milk and the honey in a saucepan (do not boil!). Then, if you prefer, froth the milk. The next step is to combine one shot of beetroot juice (or two teaspoons of beet powder), with the frothed milk and then to sprinkle with a dash of cinnamon (if desired). However, do ensure you mix the ingredients well.

<u>Quick fun fact</u>: beetroot powder can have so many different uses! Some examples are boosting the content and nutritional value of a smoothie or to add that fabulous dash of colour (in smoothies or in pancakes). It can even be used as a natural colouring (for example in the toy dough). Its health benefits are also limitless, as it is loaded with vitamins, minerals, antioxidants, dietary fibre, and nutrients. This compound, which is alkaline in nature, can give stronger blood regulation, can provide cellular healing, can increase oxygen uptake, and can provide endurance for any mechanical workouts. Pretty impressive, right?

Lunch – Roasted Vegetable and Coconut Milk Soup

This vegetable alkaline dish is very beneficial for you. The ingredients of this lunch include two cups of mixed vegetables (chopped into chunks), 20ml of extra virgin olive oil (which is used to roast vegetables), sea salt and black pepper to taste, one tablespoon of coconut oil, two cloves garlic (peeled and crushed), one tin of coconut milk and a bit of freshly grated ginger.

First and foremost, arrange the chopped vegetables in an oven-safe baking tray (drizzle with extra virgin olive oil). Then, roast in the oven at 180 degrees Celsius until soft (about 30 minutes). In the meantime, in a saucepan, heat the coconut oil and saute the garlic and ginger for a few minutes. Now, add the coconut milk and simmer for 20 minutes on medium-low heat, until reduced by a quarter. When the milk is ready, transfer it to a soup bowl and then add the roasted vegetable. Serve hot!

Day nineteen

Breakfast – Gluten-Free Berry Pie

This recipe is fantastic! It meets all the essential requirements that your body needs, such as minerals, proteins and juicy vitamins, and these all help you to yield the proper amount of energy!

To prepare this breakfast, the ingredients are: one prepared unbaked pie crust (gluten-free), fresh fruit (for example you can use 500g of strawberries and 500g of blueberries), ¼ cup of sweetener of your choice (you can use organic honey), zest and juice from half a lemon, 3 tablespoons of cornstarch, ½ cup of oats, ½ cup white rice flour, 2 tablespoons of brown sugar and 4 tablespoons of butter (melted and cooled slightly).

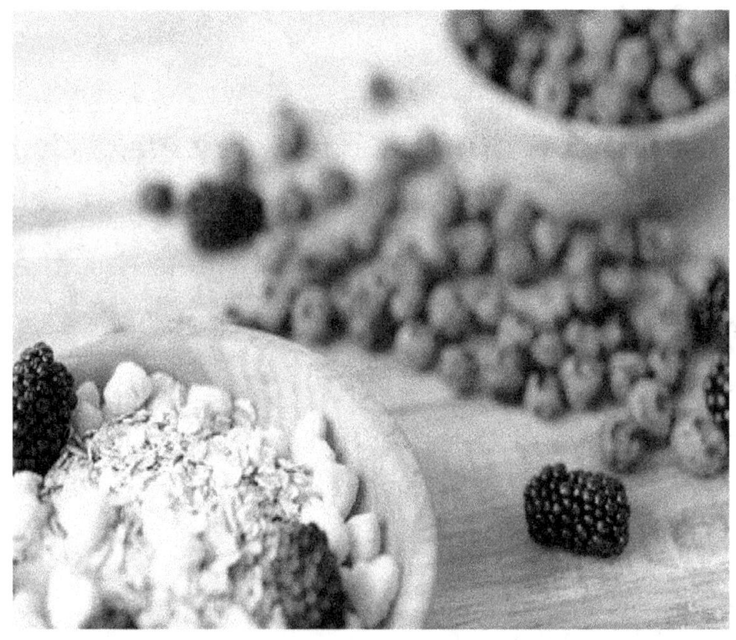

To prepare the crumb topping, you have to combine the rice flour, oats, brown sugar and melted butter in a small bowl. Then, place in the fridge (about 30 minutes). After doing this, preheat the oven to 180 degrees Celsius. The next step is to prepare the fruit: strawberries should be hulled and sliced in thick slices. Now, in a large bowl, combine the fresh fruit, honey, lemon zest, lemon juice, and cornstarch. Toss until they are well combined and then pour into the pie crust. Cover with the crumb topping. Bake in preheated oven approximately 60 minutes, until bubbling and crumb topping and pie crust are golden brown. Let cool completely before serving (you can place it in the fridge to finish cooling).

Lunch – Crunchy Quinoa Salad

This crunchy quinoa salad is perfect and delicious and it is great for your healthy state of mind. Without its use, the alkalinity of the body can easily change.

The ingredients of this salad contain one cup of uncooked quinoa, 1 1/2 cups of fresh cauliflower (chopped in pieces), extra virgin olive oil, one cucumber (sliced), one raw carrot (sliced), ½ cup of kale, 1 teaspoon of chopped fresh mint, 2 tablespoons of chopped fresh parsley, 3 tablespoons of lemon juice, a pinch of pumpkin seeds, sea salt and freshly ground black pepper.

The directions of this delicious recipe are: rinse the quinoa well and place it in a pot with water and bring to a boil. Cover and cook for 15 minutes. Remove from the heat, stir, and allow the quinoa to cool slightly.

Meanwhile, put a large pot of water on the stove to boil, drop the cauliflower and kale into the boiling water, and cook for 5 minutes, until crisp-tender (above all the cauliflower). Remove from the pot with a slotted spoon and drop into a bowl. Then drain. After doing this, combine the cooked quinoa, cauliflower, cucumber, carrot, and kale in a salad bowl. Add the remaining ingredients and mix well. Season with freshly ground black pepper and sea salt (if desired).

Day 20 - 30

For the remaining eleven days, follow a similar plan. The entire meal plan has to be similar to equate to an equal amount of intake and balance. The dinner can be anything from the dinner recipes (or from other recipes in this book), and try your best in maintaining a smaller portion.

By doing so, and following this thirty-day meal plan, you can achieve the healthy and fit body in which you are aiming for, and you can be one step closer to obtaining a proper muscle build.

Thus, it does not matter whether you are an athlete or a professional worker at all; all you need is a proper alkaline diet, and the results (having a healthy, cleaner body) will be great.

You will soon see, if you follow the diet precisely, that the results will be excellent, and you must not be afraid of giving this diet a try, because the results really will speak for themselves!

Therefore, the thirty-day meal plan is essential because it provides you with a significant amount of energy and the alkalinity, that is necessary for maintaining perfect health.

CONCLUSION

To conclude this book, you have to be very careful about your diet and what you do in your daily routine. You need to be curious about every calorie that goes in you. You have been provided with all the reasons you need to switch to an alkaline-based diet, as you have read that alkalinity can give you a healthy PH and can avert any harmful stroke of acidity in the body.

You will have read that acidity can be dangerous as it can lead to a rise in inflammatory diseases and the rupture of many digestive organs. While, on the contrary, you will have learnt that alkalinity can give you a fresh, balanced diet, full of healthy foods that will nourish, care and protect you.

The diet comes in all shapes and formats, and this book has given you breakfast recipes, lunch recipes, dinner recipes, smoothies recipes and the sweet, beautiful dessert recipes, which are sure to cause you ultimate satisfaction!

By now, I'm sure you'll realise that you do not have to be an expert in medicine to know which diet to follow. Following an alkaline diet is highly beneficial, and with all that you have read, you will be able to use these recipes to begin recovering at the earliest convenience.

These recipes have everything in their DNA. They have the minerals, the enzymes, the proteins, the amino acids. There is no rocket science behind their creation and one does not have to be very intelligent while creating them. Thus, you can follow this book and you

264

will get a splendid amount of results in no time. It is available at an affordable price.

Try your best in avoiding any acidic diet at all cost even if it gives you a great amount of relish. The idea is fats and mineral are all very delicious but they come with devious outcomes, one of them being that of fat accumulation. You need to understand that long aging is only possible if you have a balanced diet intake and this diet can be only of an alkaline nature.

To make conclusive remarks about the benefits of an alkaline diet, the first and foremost is the sheer activeness that a person tends to achieve while they are eating an alkaline diet. They feel healthy and look healthy and want to be doing a lot of things while they are enjoying an alkaline diet. They can even think properly and can get rid of inflammatory diseases that can cause them suffering. Furthermore, an alkaline diet has fantastic results in helping to brighten up your face and to make you look fresher. Studies even show how the diet is popular in making people have a healthier, more radiant face. Thus, alkalinity is very crucial for having great skin and face.

An alkaline diet also protects bone density and muscle mass, as the mineral intake that you get through an alkaline diet can protect your bone density. The bones need certain minerals that are used to cure the excessive number of hurdles one gets while running, and the minerals that are given by the alkaline diet gives you stronger bones for life. If you are a bodybuilder and want to reap the benefits, then you have to accumulate more alkaline foods, and you will soon realise that this will be extremely beneficial for you. For example, muscle mass can be secured through eating things like almonds and other alkaline foods, and you will have to be very strict in doing so. But, just look on the bright side, and tell yourself every day about the amazing health benefits you're going to get! You will soon feel incredibly productive.

In today's world, everywhere you go, you get a certain level of stress. There is the stress of graduating, the stress of succeeding in life, the stress of getting a job. You believe at first that the stress can be very successive for you and lead you on to good things, but actually, it often turns out to be adverse. Scientists have claimed medical drugs for its cure, but the only reasonable cure is the use of an alkaline diet! The enzymes that you get through vegetables lower the risk of hypertension, and then you can relish in a successful life in absolutely no time at all.

Also, your blood level starts to work with full capacity and you will feel like a superman every place you go! Therefore, it is vital you switch to an alkaline diet.

You are also able to get a lot of chronic pains in your body due to many different reasons. You get to the bottom of any problem; you solve it only to end up having chronic pain yet again in your body. Chronic pain refers to any amount of pain in your body, such as a devastating headache. However, the only effective cure for this chronic pain is the alkaline diet. Yes, it is true, the alkaline diet is very important for you to maintain as the blood level minimises when lemon or other alkaline water is introduced into the body. So, this is another benefit of an alkaline diet and it does not matter if you are a walker, a boxer or even a corporate worker, you must have an alkaline diet in you if you wish to have all that you crave!

In the end, we will only assure you good health and being a beginner, you must not waste any further time and start this diet now! Good health is wealth, and nobody became rich while being lazy and stubborn. This book is all that you need and you must follow it at all costs to ensure a healthy, better, more improved lifestyle.